Epilepsy

Editors

KAREEM A. ZAGHLOUL
EDWARD F. CHANG

NEUROSURGERY
CLINICS OF NORTH AMERICA

www.neurosurgery.theclinics.com

Consulting Editors
RUSSELL LONSER
ISAAC YANG

January 2016 • Volume 27 • Number 1

ELSEVIER

1600 John F. Kennedy Boulevard • Suite 1800 • Philadelphia, Pennsylvania, 19103-2899

http://www.theclinics.com

NEUROSURGERY CLINICS OF NORTH AMERICA Volume 27, Number 1
January 2016 ISSN 1042-3680, ISBN-13: 978-0-323-41458-6

Editor: Jennifer Flynn-Briggs
Developmental Editor: Colleen Viola

Neurosurgery Clinics of North America (ISSN 1042-3680) is published quarterly by Elsevier Inc., 360 Park Avenue South, New York, NY 10010-1710. Months of issue are January, April, July, and October. Business and Editorial Offices: 1600 John F. Kennedy Blvd., Suite 1800, Philadelphia, PA 19103-2899. Customer Service Office: 11830 Westline Industrial Drive, St. Louis, MO 63146. Periodicals postage paid at New York, NY, and additional mailing offices. Subscription prices are $385.00 per year (US individuals), $639.00 per year (US institutions), $415.00 per year (Canadian individuals), $794.00 per year (Canadian institutions), $495.00 per year (international individuals), $794.00 per year (international institutions), $100.00 per year (US students), and $255.00 per year (international and Canadian students). International air speed delivery is included in all *Clinics* subscription prices. All prices are subject to change without notice. **POSTMASTER:** Send address changes to *Neurosurgery Clinics of North America*, Elsevier Periodicals Customer Service, 11830 Westline Industrial Drive, St. Louis, MO 63146. **Customer Service: 1-800-654-2452 (US and Canada). From outside the US and Canada, call: 1-314-453-7041. Fax: 1-314-453-5170. E-mail: JournalsCustomerService-usa@elsevier.com (for print support) and journalsonlinesupport-usa@elsevier.com (for online support).**

Reprints. For copies of 100 or more, of articles in this publication, please contact the Commercial Reprints Department, Elsevier Inc., 360 Park Avenue South, New York, NY 10010-1710. Tel. 212-633-3874; Fax: 212-633-3820; E-mail: reprints@elsevier.com.

Neurosurgery Clinics of North America is covered in *MEDLINE/PubMed (Index Medicus), EMBASE/Excerpta Medica, and Current Contents/Clinical Medicine (CC/CM).*

Contributors

CONSULTING EDITORS

RUSSELL LONSER, MD
Professor and Chair, Department of
Neurological Surgery, The Ohio State
University Wexner Medical Center,
Columbus, Ohio

ISAAC YANG, MD
Attending Neurosurgeon, Assistant Professor,
Department of Neurosurgery, Director of
Medical Student Education, Jonsson
Comprehensive Cancer Center, David Geffen
School of Medicine at UCLA, University of
California Los Angeles, Los Angeles, California

EDITORS

KAREEM A. ZAGHLOUL, MD, PhD
Investigator, Surgical Neurology Branch,
National Institute of Neurological Disorders and
Stroke, National Institutes of Health, Bethesda,
Maryland

EDWARD F. CHANG, MD
Associate Professor, Department of
Neurological Surgery, University of California,
San Francisco, San Francisco, California

AUTHORS

SOHA ALOMAR, MD, MPH, FRCSC
Epilepsy Center, Neurological Institute,
Cleveland Clinic, Cleveland, Ohio

RICHARD V. ANDREWS, MD
RA Neurological, Omaha, Nebraska

S. KATHLEEN BANDT, MD
Resident Physician, Department of
Neurological Surgery, Washington
University School of Medicine, St Louis,
Missouri

NICHOLAS M. BARBARO, MD
Professor and Chair, Department of
Neurological Surgery, Indiana University,
Indianapolis, Indiana

ROBERT BUCKLEY, MD
Department of Neurological Surgery, Chief
Resident, Seattle Children's Hospital,
University of Washington, Seattle,
Washington

ANDREA JENNIFER CHAMCZUK, MD, MSc
Assistant Professor of Neurosurgery,
Creighton University Medical Center, Omaha,
Nebraska

EDWARD F. CHANG, MD
Associate Professor, Department of
Neurological Surgery, University of
California, San Francisco, San Francisco,
California

SHABBAR F. DANISH, MD
Department of Neurosurgery, Rutgers Robert
Wood Johnson Medical School, New
Brunswick, New Jersey

DANIEL L. DRANE, PhD
Associate Professor, Department of
Neurology, Emory University School of
Medicine, Atlanta, Georgia; Department
of Neurology, University of Washington
School of Medicine, Seattle, Washington

SAMUEL ESTRONZA-OJEDA, MD
Division of Neurosurgery, Research Fellow, Seattle Children's Hospital, University of Puerto Rico, San Juan, Puerto Rico

THOMAS GIANARIS, MD
Department of Neurological Surgery, Indiana University School of Medicine, Indianapolis, Indiana

JORGE GONZALEZ-MARTINEZ, MD, PhD
Epilepsy Center, Neurological Institute, Cleveland Clinic, Cleveland, Ohio

ROBERT E. GROSS, MD, PhD
MBNA/Bowman Professor of Neurosurgery, Departments of Neurosurgery and Neurology, Emory University School of Medicine; Interventional MRI Program, Emory University Hospital; Coulter Department of Biomedical Engineering, Georgia Institute of Technology, Atlanta, Georgia

CASEY HALPERN, MD
Assistant Professor of Neurosurgery and, by Courtesy, of Neurology and Neurological Sciences, and Psychiatry and Behavioral Sciences, Stanford University Medical Center, Stanford, California

KATHRYN HOES, MD, MBS
Department of Neurological Surgery, University of Texas Southwestern Medical Center, Dallas, Texas

ALASTAIR T. HOYT, MD
Department of Neurological Surgery, Barrow Neurological Institute, St. Joseph's Hospital and Medical Center, Phoenix, Arizona

JAES JONES, BS
Epilepsy Center, Neurological Institute, Cleveland Clinic, Cleveland, Ohio

NICHOLAS KON KAM KING, MD, PhD
Department of Neurosurgery, National Neuroscience Institute, Singapore

VIBHOR KRISHNA, MD, SM
Division of Neurosurgery, Toronto Western Hospital, University of Toronto, Toronto, Ontario, Canada

BRADLEY LEGA, MD
Department of Neurological Surgery, University of Texas Southwestern Medical Center, Dallas, Texas

ERIC C. LEUTHARDT, MD
Associate Professor, Department of Neurological Surgery, Washington University School of Medicine; Department of Biomedical Engineering, Washington University; Center for Innovation in Neuroscience and Technology, Washington University School of Medicine, St Louis, Missouri

ANDRES MALDONADO, MD
Epilepsy Center, Neurological Institute, Cleveland Clinic, Cleveland, Ohio

MARTHA J. MORRELL, MD
NeuroPace, Inc, Mountain View, California; Clinical Professor of Neurology and Neurological Sciences and, by Courtesy, Neurosurgery, Stanford University, Stanford, California

JEFFREY G. OJEMANN, MD
Department of Neurological Surgery, Division Chief of Neurosurgery, Seattle Children's Hospital, University of Washington, Seattle, Washington

ARUN ANGELO PATIL, MD
Professor and Chief of Neurosurgery, Creighton University Medical Center, Omaha, Nebraska

IRINA PODKORYTOVA, MD
Department of Neurology and Neurotherapeutics, University of Texas Southwestern Medical Center, Dallas, Texas

JOHN D. ROLSTON, MD, PhD
Department of Neurological Surgery, University of California, San Francisco, San Francisco, California

FRANCESCO SAMMARTINO, MD
Division of Neurosurgery, Toronto Western Hospital, University of Toronto, Toronto, Ontario, Canada

SAURABH SINHA, MD
Department of Neurosurgery, Rutgers Robert Wood Johnson Medical School, New Brunswick, New Jersey

KRIS A. SMITH, MD
Director of Gamma Knife, Department of Neurological Surgery, Barrow Neurological Institute, St. Joseph's Hospital and Medical Center, Phoenix, Arizona

ROSA QUI YUE SO, PhD
Institute for Infocomm Research, Agency for Science, Technology and Research, Singapore

RICHARD WENNBERG, MD, PhD
Division of Neurology, Krembil Neuroscience Centre, Toronto Western Hospital, University Health Network, Professor, University of Toronto, Toronto, Ontario, Canada

JON T. WILLIE, MD, PhD
Assistant Professor, Departments of Neurosurgery and Neurology, Emory University School of Medicine; Interventional MRI Program, Emory University Hospital, Atlanta, Georgia

THOMAS WITT, MD
Department of Neurological Surgery, Indiana University Health, Indianapolis, Indiana

ROSA QUI YUE SO, PhD
Institute for Infocomm Research, Agency for Science, Technology and Research, Singapore

RICHARD WENNBERG, MD, PhD
Division of Neurology, Krembil Neuroscience Centre, Toronto Western Hospital, University Health Network, Professor, University of Toronto, Toronto, Ontario, Canada

JOHN T. WILLIE, MD, PhD
Assistant Professor, Departments of Neurosurgery and Neurology, Emory University School of Medicine, Interventional MRI Program, Emory University Hospital, Atlanta, Georgia

THOMAS WITT, MD
Department of Neurological Surgery, Indiana University Health, Indianapolis, Indiana

Contents

> Mesial temporal lobe epilepsy is a common condition that is frequently drug resistant. Anterior temporal lobectomy has been shown to be effective in controlling seizures but entails resecting anterior and lateral temporal lobe regions that are not necessarily included in the epileptogenic zone. Selective amygdalohippocampectomy spares uninvolved structures while providing the same benefit as anterior temporal lobectomy. This article describes the three most common surgical approaches for performing selective amygdalohippocampectomy and discusses their relative merits and risks.

> Multiple hippocampal transection (MHT) is a novel surgical procedure that serves to disrupt seizure propagation fibers within the hippocampus without impairing verbal memory or the loss of stem cells. Given the paucity of literature regarding the utility and long-term outcome of MHT, a review is presented of the current literature to support the utility of this procedure in the treatment of intractable temporal lobe epilepsy. Long-term outcome analysis of this technique has been reported by two independent groups. Both groups used intraoperative electrocorticography. All patients underwent multiple subpial transection on the neocortex and MHT on the hippocampus.

> The history of epilepsy surgery is generally noted to have begun in 1886 with Victor Horsley's first report of craniotomies for posttraumatic epilepsy. With increased understanding of brain function and development of electroencephalographic methods, nonlesional epilepsy began to be treated with resection in the 1950s. Methodological improvements and increased understanding of pathophysiology followed, and the advent of stereotaxy and ablative technology in the 1960s and 1970s heralded a new era of minimally invasive, targeted procedures for lesional and nonlesional epilepsy. Current techniques combine stereotactic methods, improved ablative technologies, and electroencephalographic methods for a multidisciplinary approach to the neurosurgical treatment of epilepsy.

 Video of laser ablation accompanies this article

> Stereotactic laser amygdalohippocampotomy (SLAH) uses laser interstitial thermal therapy guided by magnetic resonance thermography. This novel intervention can

of open surgery's associated risks. By evading these risks, they also open up treatment options to patients who otherwise are poor surgical candidates. Radiosurgery is one of the most intensively studied of these alternatives and has found a growing role in the treatment of medial temporal lobe epilepsy.

nonresponsive therapeutic neurostimulation. Currently, the main modalities in clinical use, from most invasive to least invasive, are anterior thalamus deep brain stimulation, vagus nerve stimulation, and trigeminal nerve stimulation. Significant reductions in seizure frequency have been demonstrated in clinical trials using each of these neuromodulation therapies.

NEUROSURGERY CLINICS OF NORTH AMERICA

FORTHCOMING ISSUES

April 2016
Meningiomas
Gabriel Zada and Randy L. Jensen, *Editors*

July 2016
Trigeminal Neuralgia
John Y.K. Lee and Michael Lim, *Editors*

October 2016
Traumatic Brain Injury
Daniel Hirt, Paul Vespa, and Geoffrey Manley, *Editors*

RECENT ISSUES

October 2015
Chiari Malformation
Jeffrey Leonard and David Limbrick, *Editors*

July 2015
Endoscopic Endonasal Skull Base Surgery
Daniel M. Prevedello, *Editor*

April 2015
Quality Improvement in Neurosurgery
John D. Rolston, Seunggu J. Han, and Andrew T. Parsa, *Editors*

RELATED INTEREST

Pediatric Clinics, June 2015 (Vol. 62, Issue 3)
New Advances in Pediatric Neurologic and Developmental Disorders in the Era of Genomics
Gyula Acsadi, *Editor*

THE CLINICS ARE AVAILABLE ONLINE!
Access your subscription at:
www.theclinics.com

NEUROSURGERY CLINICS OF NORTH AMERICA

Preface
Minimally Invasive Epilepsy Surgery

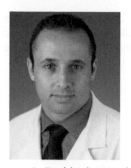
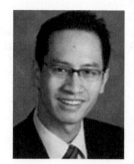

Kareem A. Zaghloul, MD, PhD   Edward F. Chang, MD

Editors

Refractory seizures in patients with epilepsy are associated with significant morbidity, cognitive decline, and premature death. For many patients, surgery may be the most promising option for becoming seizure free. As such, both the American Academy of Neurology and the American Association of Neurological Surgeons have released guidelines recommending a comprehensive evaluation for surgery in patients with medically refractory epilepsy.

The potential benefits of surgical intervention in patients with medically refractory epilepsy have been clearly established, particularly for patients with temporal lobe epilepsy. Class I evidence has demonstrated that anterior temporal lobectomy is superior to medical management in obtaining seizure freedom in patients with mesial temporal sclerosis. Multiple studies have supported these findings and have shown that surgical resection in these patients can result in seizure-freedom rates up to 60% to 80% after 2 years, and up to 50% at 10 years following surgery.

Unfortunately, despite the potential benefits offered by surgical intervention in patients with medically refractory epilepsy, surgery is vastly underutilized. There are a number of possible reasons for this. Despite the fact that many studies have documented the relatively low morbidity of epilepsy surgery, it is still largely viewed as an invasive and risky treatment option among epileptologists and neurologists and is often only recommended as a treatment of last resort. Furthermore, particularly in cases of extratemporal lobe epilepsy, the benefits of surgery are still not clearly established. In these cases, surgical intervention may actually require two procedures, one for the placement of intracranial electrodes for proper localization of seizure activity and identification of eloquent cortex and a second for resection of epileptogenic tissue. Hence, in these cases, there is additional risk, without guaranteed benefit.

In this special issue of the *Neurosurgery Clinics of North America*, we have chosen to highlight recent advances in epilepsy surgery that begin to address these outstanding issues and concerns. We have curated a collection of articles from respected leaders of the field presenting their work describing minimally invasive surgical techniques for epilepsy. Although broadly grouped together under this common theme, the articles selected here in fact span minimally invasive open surgical procedures, ablative procedures, shifting trends in invasive monitoring, and the role of neuromodulation for epilepsy. These approaches represent exciting and novel developments in epilepsy surgery aimed at minimizing the associated morbidities of surgical intervention while capitalizing on surgery's potential benefits for patients with medically refractory epilepsy.

Kareem A. Zaghloul, MD, PhD
Surgical Neurology Branch
National Institute of Neurological
Disorders and Stroke, NIH
Building 10, Room 3D20
10 Center Drive
Bethesda, MD 20892-1414, USA

Edward F. Chang, MD
Department of Neurological Surgery
University of California
San Francisco
505 Parnassus Avenue, M-779
San Francisco, CA 94143-0112, USA

E-mail addresses:
kareem.zaghloul@nih.gov (K.A. Zaghloul)
Edward.Chang@ucsf.edu (E.F. Chang)

Selective Amygdalohippocampectomy

Alastair T. Hoyt, MD, Kris A. Smith, MD*

KEYWORDS

- Amygdalohippocampectomy • Epilepsy • Mesial temporal sclerosis • Subtemporal
- Temporal lobectomy • Transcortical • Transsylvian

KEY POINTS

- Selective amygdalohippocampectomy effectively reduces seizure severity and frequency in patients with mesial temporal epilepsy.
- Selective procedures seem to be as effective as anterior temporal lobectomy in patients whose disease is limited to the mesial temporal structures.
- Although the evidence is inconclusive, it suggests that selective amygdalohippocampectomy may preserve neurocognitive function better than anterior temporal lobectomy.
- Multiple approaches are available to access the mesial temporal structures.
- There is no definitive evidence for the superiority of a particular approach in terms of seizure control or neurocognitive outcome.

INTRODUCTION

Eliminating seizures while preserving a patient's neurologic function is the defining goal of all epilepsy surgery. Epilepsy of the temporal lobe, and specifically epilepsy localized to the mesial temporal structures, is by far the most common focal epilepsy in adults and is among the most common focal epilepsies afflicting children.[1] Mesial temporal lobe epilepsy (MTLE) is also among the least likely type of epilepsy to be adequately controlled with medical treatment alone.[2] A prospective randomized controlled trial published by Wiebe and colleagues[3] demonstrated that anterior temporal lobectomy (ATL) with resection of the mesial temporal structures is superior to medical management for drug-resistant MTLE. Engel and colleagues[4] confirmed their findings in 2012 in a similarly methodologically sound study. Such resection offers increased quality of life to patients[5] and has been found to be cost-effective in both children and adults.[6–8]

However, anteromedial temporal lobe resection entails resection of the anterior portion of the temporal lobe, which may not be implicated in seizure production in isolated mesial temporal disease. Driven by a desire to preserve structures outside of the epileptogenic zone, investigators have developed so-called selective procedures. Specifically, selective amygdalohippocampectomy (SAHC) has been described as an alternative to target only the mesial temporal structures while preserving the lateral neocortex, temporal pole, and temporal white matter tracts.[9–11] No incontrovertible evidence exists, but selective procedures should theoretically reduce the morbidity of epilepsy surgery.[12]

Although the terms *ATL* and *SAHC* are commonly used for this procedure, both terms are somewhat misleading. As described by most investigators, ATL involves resection of not only the anterior portion of the temporal lobe but also most of the hippocampus, amygdala, and parahippocampal structures. Similarly, SAHC involves

Disclosures: The authors have no financial disclosures.
Department of Neurological Surgery, Barrow Neurological Institute, St. Joseph's Hospital and Medical Center, 350 West Thomas Road, Phoenix, AZ 85013, USA
* Corresponding author.
E-mail address: neuropub@dignityhealth.org

neurosurgery.theclinics.com

resection of the bulk of the hippocampus, amygdala, and parahippocampal structures.

PATIENT EVALUATION OVERVIEW
Indications

SAHC is reserved for patients with disabling, medically intractable seizures that originate unilaterally in mesial temporal structures (**Box 1**).[4,13–15] The American Academy of Neurology recommends that patients with drug-resistant MTLE resulting in disabling complex partial seizures be referred for surgery[5] because of a single randomized controlled trial and a further 24 observational studies.[16] The International League Against Epilepsy (ILAE) defined drug resistance as failure of 2 tolerated, appropriately chosen, and used antiepileptic drug schedules.[15]

Preoperative Evaluation

There are 2 key factors in selecting a patient for SAHC. First, localization of the epileptogenic zone to the mesial temporal structures is paramount. Second, assessment of the risk for function decline due to surgery is no less important. A full discussion of seizure localization and risk assessment is beyond the scope of this article, but most investigators[2,16–20] agree that a thorough neurologic examination, clear understanding of the seizure semiology, interictal electroencephalographic (EEG) evaluation, high-resolution magnetic resonance imaging (MRI) of the brain, and neuropsychological evaluation represent a minimum presurgical investigation (**Box 2**). Indeed, the ILAE Subcommission for Pediatric Epilepsy Surgery concluded that interictal EEG, neuropsychological assessment, and high-resolution MRI were mandatory.[19]

Box 1
Patient selection for SAHC

Indications
- Disabling, drug-resistant, mesial temporal lobe epilepsy

Contraindications
- Evidence that patients will have neurocognitive decline with surgery, which would outweigh the benefit of seizure control
- Multifocal onset of seizures or bilateral independent mesial temporal lobe onset
- Patients' general medical inability to tolerate surgery

Abbreviations: SAHC, selective amygdalohippocampectomy.

Box 2
Presurgical epilepsy evaluation

Mandatory studies
- Review of seizure history, semiology, and symptoms
- Neuropsychological evaluation
- Video scalp EEG monitoring
- High-resolution MRI with coronal projections

Complementary studies
- PET with fludeoxyglucose F 18
- Ictal single-photon emission computed tomography
- Magnetoencephalography
- Intracarotid amobarbital testing (Wada test)
- Selective posterior cerebral artery amobarbital testing (selective Wada test)
- Intracranial EEG electrode monitoring
- Functional MRI
- Diffusion tensor imaging

Abbreviations: EEG, electroencephalography; MRI, magnetic resonance imaging; PET, positron emission tomography.

Complementary evaluation techniques can also be of great value. However, a well-designed systematic review by Burch and colleagues[21] of noninvasive presurgical evaluation other than EEG and MRI identified no randomized trials or cohort studies, and minimal high-quality evidence of effectiveness in any individual complementary study. The investigators opined that each of the complementary techniques may be useful in the context of a comprehensive evaluation and recommended thorough discussion of individual cases in a multidisciplinary conference to provide an optimal surgical plan. As elegantly described by Spencer and Burchiel,[20] the selection of patients should depend on converging lines of evidence.

Some investigators advocate reserving SAHC for cases when imaging abnormalities are present on MRI.[13] Other surgeons argue that if there is reasonable confidence of a mesial temporal seizure origin, SAHC may be offered with the option of completing resection of the neocortical structures at a later date if necessary. ATL with resection of the medial structures may be more appropriate if there are findings consistent with neocortical sources.[22] The senior author's current practice is to stereotactically implant depth electrodes into the hippocampus and amygdala bilaterally in MRI-negative patients in order to ensure unilateral, medial-onset seizures before offering SAHC. Preponderant unilateral magnetoencephalograph spikes may be an alternative noninvasive confirmatory test; however, there are currently only limited data to support this practice.[23]

Timing of Surgery

The Early Randomized Surgical Epilepsy Trial results suggest that patients with MTLE benefit from early intervention.[4] In that study, patients with MTLE, hippocampal sclerosis, and disabling drug-resistant seizures for less than 2 years were randomized to surgery or medical treatment. None of the 23 patients in the medical group and 11 of 15 patients in the surgical group were seizure free at the 2-year follow-up. Unpublished data from the authors' center (KA Smith, 2012) suggests that surgical treatment (lesionectomy without SAHC) of patients who are discovered to have cavernous malformations of the mesial temporal structures within 6 months of the onset of seizures results in superior seizure control outcomes relative to patients who have been treated medically for more than 1 year before surgery.

Despite these findings, studies suggest that many patients present for surgical evaluation only after many years of symptoms. At Columbia University in New York, the mean duration from the onset of symptoms to referral to a comprehensive epilepsy program was 22.6 years from 1996 to 1999 and 21.1 years from 2004 to 2007.[24] At the University of California, Los Angeles, the mean duration was 17.1 years from 1995 to 1998 and 18.6 years from 2005 to 2008.[25]

Patient Age

There is some evidence to suggest that pediatric patients respond differently than adult patients to SAHC.[13] Clusmann and colleagues[26] compared ATL and SAHC in a pediatric cohort and found that 94% of patients obtained a good outcome (Engel classes I and II) with ATL compared with 74% with SAHC. Datta and colleagues[27] compared the outcome after SAHC in an adult and pediatric cohort and found superior outcomes in the adult patient population, with 100% of the treated adults and only 55% of the treated children achieving Engel class I and II outcomes. The pathophysiological basis for these observations remains unclear.[13] The authors speculate that the pediatric population of patients with refractory epilepsy includes a higher percentage of patients with congenital abnormalities in the temporal lobe or genetically based primary epilepsies as compared with the typically acquired MTLE seen in adults.

SURGICAL TREATMENT OPTIONS

Many approaches to the mesial temporal structures have been described.[9,13,28–43] The 3 best described methods among these approaches are the transcortical, transsylvian, and subtemporal approaches. A brief history, surgical details, and special considerations of each approach are discussed in the order in which they were first described in the literature.

Transcortical Approach

Overview
Niemeyer[43] first described the transventricular amygdalohippocampectomy in 1958. The approach he described has subsequently been termed the transcortical SAHC (TC SAHC). In 1969, Niemeyer and Bello[35] described the same approach using microsurgical techniques. In the original description, the temporal lobe was entered in the middle temporal gyrus. Other investigators have described modifications of this technique with access through the superior temporal gyrus,[20] superior temporal sulcus,[44] middle temporal gyrus,[13,37] and inferior temporal sulcus.[38] Regardless of the exact site of access to the temporal lobe, this approach traverses the lateral temporal structures to provide access to the temporal horn of the lateral ventricle and, thus, the amygdala, hippocampus, and parahippocampal gyrus. Variations have also been developed using multiple cranial exposures, including a limited temporal craniotomy[38] and a small keyhole craniotomy centered over the middle temporal gyrus.[45]

Operative procedure
Patients are positioned either in a lateral decubitus position or supine with the shoulder ipsilateral to the surgical site elevated. The head is fixated and rotated contralateral such that the axis of the temporal lobe lies horizontally. A pretragal linear incision[37,46] or a curvilinear frontotemporal incision[13] based just above the zygoma is opened and the temporalis is divided. Stereotactic navigation can be very helpful in planning a craniotomy, particularly if a small craniotomy is planned that does not provide complete visualization of the lateral temporal anatomy.[13,38,45,46] A corticotomy is performed and extended to a length of 2 to 3 cm parallel to the superior temporal sulcus. Dissection is carried medially under microscopic magnification, splitting the white matter fibers in a slitlike fashion in the anteroposterior direction, until the temporal horn of the lateral ventricle is encountered. Self-retaining retractors are then frequently placed to maintain the working corridor. The hippocampus, choroid plexus, choroidal

fissure, and amygdala can be visualized on the medial inferior walls of the ventricle.

An opening is made in the ependyma at the ventricular sulcus at the junction of the hippocampus and the collateral eminence, and dissection is carried into the parahippocampal gyrus. With a combination of microdissection and ultrasonic aspiration, a subpial dissection of the parahippocampal gyrus in performed. The tentorial edge, oculomotor nerve, posterior communicating artery, posterior cerebral artery, and optic tract are typically visible through the pia; care should be taken to not violate the pia to preserve these structures. Subpial dissection is carried forward into the tissue of the uncus. With traction from microdissectors, the choroidal fissure can be opened and the thin attachment of the fimbria hippocampi can be divided, allowing the hippocampus to be mobilized laterally and inferiorly. The vessels of the hippocampal arcade are coagulated and divided as close as possible to the hippocampus to avoid injury to the parent vessels. The hippocampus is transected in the coronal plane at the junction of the body and tail, providing an en bloc resection of the body and head of the hippocampus.

Attention is turned to the residual parahippocampal gyrus and amygdala, which is resected within the bounds of the medial and inferior pial margins. The amygdala may be as high as the horizontal segment of the middle cerebral artery (MCA). Additional subpial ultrasonic aspiration and microdissection of the tail of the hippocampus is carried posteriorly from the site of the coronal transection to at least the plane of the colliculi. The wound is irrigated and closed.

Special surgical considerations
The location of the lateral temporal corticotomy can be varied, depending on the required angle to approach the mesial structures on navigation.[13] Some investigators[37] advocate placing the incision in a more posterior position (just anterior to the plane of the central sulcus) in the nondominant hemisphere and in a more anterior position (just anterior to the plane of the precentral sulcus) in the dominant hemisphere. The use of intraoperative image-guided navigation can also be used to tailor an entry site.[45,47]

Transsylvian Approach

Overview
The transsylvian approach for SAHC (TS SAHC) was introduced by Yaşargil and colleagues in 1973 and was first described by Wieser and Yaşargil[48] in 1982, with several subsequent descriptions.[10,11,39] Various investigators have now

described variations on the approach.[2,49,50] This approach takes advantage of the sylvian fissure to access the mesial temporal region without disruption of the lateral and anterior neocortex of the white matter tracts surrounding the lateral ventricle. Yaşargil and colleagues' stated goal was to perform a "pure lesionectomy."[11]

Operative procedure
Patients are positioned in the supine position with the shoulder ipsilateral to the operative site supported. The head is fixated and rotated such that the malar eminence is the highest point of the surgical field to bring the sylvian fissure into a roughly vertical orientation. A semilunar incision is opened similar to other pterional approaches. The temporalis may be divided or dissected via an interfascial technique. A craniotomy is fashioned overlying the sylvian fissure. The craniotomy should extend superior to the fissure by approximately 1.5 cm. A drill is used to flatten the greater and lesser wings of the sphenoid to the level of the superior orbital fissure to facilitate exposure. The dura is opened and reflected over the remolded sphenoid and orbit. Under microscopic magnification, the sylvian fissure is opened from the region of the carotid bifurcation to about 2 cm distal to the MCA bifurcation. The limen insulae, ascending M1 branch, and anterior third of the insular cortex with its associated M2 branches can be visualized. The inferior circular sulcus, which separates the temporal operculum from the insula, is identified.

A 1- to 2-cm corticotomy is created in the temporal stem at the level of the limen insulae, and dissection is carried down to the uncus parallel to the M1 segment until the temporal horn of the lateral ventricle is encountered. The tissue within the uncus is resected by subpial dissection, taking care that the pia-arachnoid boundary is left intact. The amygdala can be identified at the anterior border of a line between the choroidal fissure and the limen insulae. The amygdala and associated entorhinal cortex in the anterior portion of the parahippocampal gyrus are resected. The opening into the ventricle is extended posteriorly to better visualize the choroid emerging from the choroidal fissure, which will mark the mesial boundary of hippocampal dissection. An incision is created in the floor of the lateral ventricle, lateral to the hippocampus in the region of the collateral eminence, and carried down to the collateral sulcus. This incision defines the lateral boundary of the resection. Microdissectors and gentle traction are used to define the superior medial border of the hippocampus along the choroidal fissure. This incision provides access to the hippocampal vessels entering the hippocampal fissure, which are divided as closely as possible to the hippo-campus to avoid injury to the parent vessels. Sub-pial dissection is carried along the pial boarder of the subiculum and the inferior parahippocampal gyrus until it meets with the lateral portion of the dissection near the collateral sulcus. The body of the hippocampus and the associated parahippo-campal gyrus are then transected in the coronal plane as posteriorly in the exposure as possible, resulting in an en bloc resection of the hippocam-pus and parahippocampal gyrus. Additional resec-tion of the tail of the hippocampus may be pursed with ultrasonic aspiration to ensure that the poste-rior extent of resection reaches the tectal plate. The wound is irrigated and closed in a typical fashion.

Special surgical considerations

The narrow working corridor of the transsylvian route requires the surgeon to be familiar with the surgical anatomy and handling of the vascular structures. Meticulous handling of the sylvian veins is essential, and medial mobilization of the MCA's temporal trunk may provide additional space for cortical incision. A generous opening of the fissure is thought to be key to avoiding vascular complications.[2]

Subtemporal Approach

Overview

Several investigators, including Hori and col-leagues,[42] Park and colleagues,[40] and Takaya and colleagues,[41] have described SAHC via a sub-temporal corridor (ST SAHC). The subtemporal approach avoids disruption of the neocortical tis-sue of the lateral temporal lobe and the white mat-ter pathways, which traverse the periventricular white matter and temporal stem. The authors favor a minimal access approach, which carries the additional advantages of a small craniotomy and small wound (**Figs. 1** and **2**).[9]

Operative procedure

Patients are positioned supine with a large shoul-der roll placed under the ipsilateral shoulder. The head is secured in a head holder, rotated contralat-eral to the operative side, and placed in lateral extension such that the zygoma is the highest point of the surgical field. The surgeon remains posi-tioned at the vertex throughout the procedure. Mannitol and modest hyperventilation are given to aid in brain relaxation. A 4- to 5-cm pretragal inci-sion is opened based at the zygoma and extending curving posteriorly just above the pinna. The tem-poralis is divided, and fishhooks are placed to retract soft tissue and maintain a low profile in the field. Stereotactic guidance is used to identify the

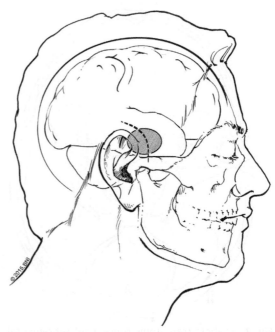

Fig. 1. Stereotactic keyhole temporal approach showing curved incision (*dashed line*) and approxi-mate position of the small craniotomy allowing access to the floor of the middle fossa for subtemporal amygdalohippocampectomy. (*Courtesy of* Barrow Neurological Institute, Phoenix, AZ; with permission.)

temporal floor, where a small burr hole is made in the inferior aspect of the exposure. An ovoid crani-otomy measuring approximately 2.5 cm in diam-eter is fashioned based on the temporal floor. It is often helpful to widen and flatten the inferior aspect of the cranial opening with a high-speed drill to bring the inferior margin of the craniotomy flush with the temporal floor and provide a slightly wider working corridor. Reverse Trendelenburg posi-tioning is used initially to aid in brain relaxation.

The operating microscope is introduced. The dura mater is opened revealing the inferior tempo-ral gyrus. A wide nonstick Cottonoid is introduced beneath the inferior temporal gyrus, and cerebro-spinal fluid is aspirated from the extra-axial space to aid in relaxation. Working along the inferior aspect of the temporal lobe, the collateral sulcus is identified. Stereotactic guidance is used to establish a trajectory to the tip of the temporal horn of the lateral ventricle. A small corticotomy is opened in the lateral inferior aspect of the para-hippocampal gyrus after opening the collateral sul-cus; dissection is carried into the uncus, gradually aiming progressively cephalad. The floor of the lateral temporal horn of the lateral ventricle is opened near its tip and extended posteriorly. This position provides visualization of the land-marks on the medial wall of the ventricle important

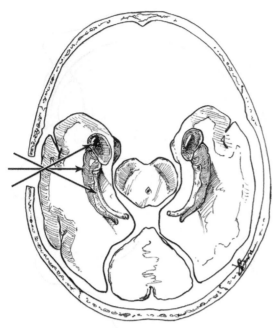

Fig. 2. Keyhole craniotomy concept for subtemporal amygdalohippocampectomy. The craniotomy is based on the temporal floor (*middle arrow*). To reach the amygdala, patients are rotated and the operating microscope is angled anteriorly (*top arrow*). To reach the tail of the hippocampus, patients are rotated in the opposite direction and the microscope is angled posteriorly (*bottom arrow*). (*From* Little AS, Smith KA, Kirlin K, et al. Modifications to the subtemporal selective amygdalohippocampectomy using a minimal-access technique: seizure and neuropsychological outcomes. J Neurosurg 2009;111(6):1272; with permission.)

to guiding the remainder of the resection, which are familiar from the TC SAHC or ATL.

The posterior inferior surface of the amygdala is identified just anterior and superior to the choroid plexus arising from the choroidal fissure. The amygdala is resected with ultrasonic aspiration until the pial surface adjacent to the sylvian fissure is identified, thereby defining the superior and anterior limits of amygdala resection. Subpial dissection with microdissectors is carried along this boundary until the remaining uncal tissue is resected. The tentorial edge, oculomotor nerve, posterior communicating artery, posterior cerebral artery, and optic tract are typically visible through the pia.

After completion of the amygdalectomy, attention is turned to the hippocampus. A Cottonoid is placed along the superior margin of the choroid plexus at the body of the hippocampus. Countertraction is placed against the Cottonoid as microdissectors are used to peel the hippocampus inferiorly from the choroidal fissure. This plane is developed posteriorly, and the hippocampus is transected in the coronal plane with ultrasonic

aspiration extending to the inferior medial pial margin. Working anteriorly from the transection of the hippocampus, the surgeon elevates the parahippocampal gyrus from the pia. The parahippocampal tissue at the head of the hippocampus is likewise elevated from the medial and inferior pial boundaries. At this juncture, the hippocampus is tethered only by the arcade of vessels entering the hippocampal fissure. These vessels are coagulated and divided as closely to the hippocampus as possible. The head and body of the hippocampus may be removed en bloc.

Attention is turned to the tail of the hippocampus posterior to the site of the coronal transection. The tail is aspirated ultrasonically beyond the level of the tectal plate into the atrium. The remaining parahippocampal gyrus is likewise resected to the pial reflection at the medial temporal-occipital junction. The wound is irrigated until complete hemostasis is ensured and then is closed. Postoperative MRI is routinely performed to assess for any retraction injury and to document the extent of hippocampal resection back to the level of the tectal plate (**Fig. 3**).

Special surgical considerations

Care should be taken to preserve the basal surface of the temporal lobe and to minimize retraction, particularly in the lateral aspect of the exposure traversed by large anastomotic veins. These veins, if present, are not retracted to prevent avulsion. Although self-retaining retractors can be placed to aid in elevation of the temporal lobe, this is typically not necessary and is avoided to prevent retraction injury. Initially placing patients in the reverse Trendelenburg position with continued cerebrospinal fluid aspiration allows development of the subtemporal space, and gradual progression to a slight Trendelenburg position allows for the upward angle necessary for access to the mesial structures. Working instruments may be used for dynamic retraction during the procedure as needed. Frequent repositioning of the head and microscope with the aid of intraoperative image guidance allows access with minimal retraction, and patients should be firmly secured to the operating table to prevent intraoperative movement.

Other Approaches

A variety of other approaches for SAHC have been described (**Table 1**). Vajkoczy and colleagues[28] described a transsylvian-transcisternal approach, which involved opening of the chiasmatic, carotid, interpeduncular, and ambient cisterns via a transsylvian exposure to mobilize the medial surface of the temporal lobe. Figueiredo and colleagues[29] described a mini-modified orbitozygomatic

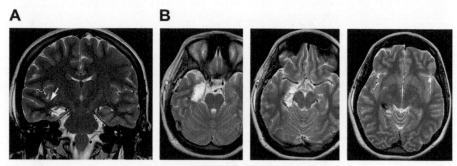

Fig. 3. (*A*) Postoperative coronal T2-weighted magnetic resonance imaging (MRI) showing that the hippocampus was resected with preservation of all lateral temporal lobe structures. The approach does not disrupt the temporal stem (*arrow*). (*B*) Postoperative axial T2-weighted MRI obtained at different levels showing selective resection of the mesial temporal structures. The hippocampus was resected posteriorly just beyond the level of the collicular plate. (*From* Little AS, Smith KA, Kirlin K, et al. Modifications to the subtemporal selective amygdalohippocampectomy using a minimal-access technique: seizure and neuropsychological outcomes. J Neurosurg 2009;111(6):1269; with permission.)

approach to the mesial temporal structures through a small supraorbital craniotomy in a cadaveric study, proposing that an anterior approach would theoretically preserve the lateral temporal cortex, lateral basal cortex, temporal stem, and optic tract. Similarly, Chen and colleagues[30] described a transorbital endoscopic approach in cadaveric specimens. Türe and colleagues[31] described approaching the mesial temporal structures from the posterior aspect via a supracerebellar-transtentorial approach.[32] Shimizu and colleagues[33] outlined a subtemporal zygomatic approach, and Miyamoto and colleagues[34] described a subtemporal and transventricular/transchoroidal approach. **Fig. 4** illustrates the general differences between the various approaches to the mesial temporal structures.

SURGICAL COMPLICATIONS

Avoidance of complications during and after SAHC is of the utmost importance because many patients are neurologically intact.[1] The surgeon and patients should undertake a detailed discussion of risks, benefits, and alternatives before surgery. Clear estimation of risks is difficult, partially because some ill effects of surgery, such as visual field defects, have at times been considered expected, inevitable, or acceptable.[1,51]

In a structured review of the literature in 2013, Georgiadis and colleagues[1] identified reported complications in adult and pediatric patients undergoing resective temporal lobe surgeries. Only 2 studies in the group focused exclusively on SAHC. In addition, individual reports of surgical

Table 1
Theoretical advantages of various approaches to SAHC

Approach	Transcortical	Transsylvian	Subtemporal
Advantages	• Can be performed with a minimal access craniotomy and small wound • Provides good visualization of ventricular and medial temporal anatomy	• Avoids injury to lateral temporal neocortex • Avoids injury to white matter tracts lateral to the temporal horn • Provides good visualization of ventricular and medial temporal anatomy	• Avoids injury to lateral temporal neocortex • Avoids injury to temporal white matter tracts and the temporal stem • Can be performed with a minimal-access craniotomy and small wound
Disadvantages	• Requires incision of lateral temporal neocortex • Disrupts white matter tracts lateral to the ventricle	• Requires a substantial craniotomy • Entails the incumbent risks of transsylvian dissection • Requires incision of the temporal stem	• Small working corridor • Visualization of anatomy can be challenging • Requires some retraction of the basal temporal lobe and possible traction on the vein of Labbé

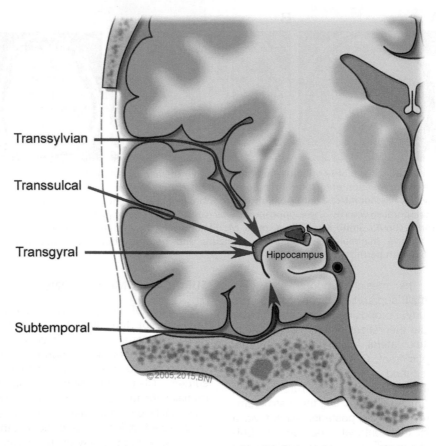

Transsylvian

Transsulcal

Transgyral

Hippocampus

Subtemporal

©2005,2015,BNI

Fig. 4. The different approaches to the hippocampus. Note that the transsylvian approach involves some transection of the temporal stem in order to gain access to the temporal horn and visualize the hippocampus. The transsulcal and trans-T2–gyral approaches are technically easiest to perform; however, they result in injury and some disconnection of the lateral temporal white matter in order to access the mesial structures. The subtemporal approach, by entering into the collateral sulcus between the fusiform and parahippocampal gyrus, spares all of the lateral temporal structures and the frontotemporal connections of the temporal stem and, therefore, should theoretically have potentially the best chance of preserving cognitive functions related to the lateral temporal lobe. (*Courtesy of* Barrow Neurological Institute, Phoenix, AZ; with permission.)

complications after SAHC can be identified in the literature (**Table 2**). No deaths as a result of surgery were noted.

Jobst and Cascino[52] systematically reviewed 55 publications from 1993 to 2014. When temporal lobe operations including ALT were included, a mortality rate of 0.4% was reported. Transient neurologic complications occurred in approximately 10% of patients, and permanent neurologic complications were noted in about 5%. One-half of the permanent deficits were visual field defects. Major complications, such as infarction and hydrocephalus, occurred in 1.5%, whereas minor complications occurred in 5%. The most frequently reported minor complications were cerebrospinal fluid leak (8.5%), aseptic meningitis (3.6%), wound infections (3%), and hemorrhage (2.5%). Separately, an inpatient database of complication rates for ATL showed an 8% overall incidence.[53]

Ischemic Events

Engel and colleagues[4] reported that 21.4% of patients demonstrated ischemic changes following SAHC on postoperative MRI imaging, but only 7.1% were symptomatic because of these changes. There is evidence of increased blood flow velocities after TS SAHC,[54,55] but it is unclear if this represents symptomatic vasospasm. Martens and colleagues[56] reported a 47.9% rate of temporal lobe infarcts and a 10.4% rate of frontal lobe infarcts after TS SAHC. Interestingly, none of the infarcts led to clinical symptoms, and patients with infarcts were more often seizure free following surgery. Neuropsychological study of those patients showed that in language-dominant hemisphere temporal lobe infarcts, verbal memory performance suffered but verbal fluency and speech comprehension were not significantly affected.

Table 2
Select publications detailing surgical complications after SAHC

Author, Year	Approach	Study Design	Number of Patients	Complications Reported	Notes
Vajkoczy et al,[28] 1998	Modified TS SAHC	Retrospective	32	Epidural/subdural hematoma 6% CN III palsy 9% VFD 3%	Perimetry was performed on 93% of patients. CN palsy was transient in all cases.
Oertel et al,[106] 2004	TC SAHC	Prospective	60	Hemiparesis 5% CN palsy 5% Aphasia 1.7% Infection 1.7%	The use of intraoperative navigation on complications was compared: 7.9% with navigation and 21.7% without.
Hori et al,[101] 2007	ST SAHC	Retrospective	26	VFD 7%	Visual field testing was performed in only 10 patients.
Acar et al,[107] 2008	TC SAHC	Retrospective	39	VFD 10.3% Aphasia 2.6% Hemiparesis 2.6% CN palsy 2.6% Hemotympanum 2.6% Frontal branch of facial nerve palsy 2.6%	Hemiparesis, CN palsy, and aphasia were all transient.
Tanriverdi et al,[62] 2008	TC SAHC	Retrospective	50	VFD 2%	Visual field testing was not performed.
Little et al,[9] 2009	ST SAHC	Retrospective	36	Frontal branch of facial nerve palsy 3% VFD 3%	Visual field testing was done by confrontation.
Yaşargil et al,[11] 2010	TS SAHC	Retrospective	73	Aphasia 11% Subdural hematoma 1.3% VFD 1.3% CN III palsy 4%	Speech disturbance and CN III palsy were transient in all patients.
Bandt et al,[108] 2013	TC SAHC	Retrospective	76	Transient aphasia 2.7%	Visual field testing was not performed.

Abbreviations: CN, cranial nerve; SAHC, selective amygdalohippocampectomy; ST SAHC, subtemporal SAHC; TC SAHC, transcortical SAHC; TS SAHC, transsylvian SAHC; VFD, visual field defect.
Data from Refs.[9,11,28,62,101,106–108]

Visual Field Deficits

The anterior bundle of the geniculocalcarine tract makes a prominent anterior curve, known as the Meyer loop, and traverses the temporal lobe in the roof and lateral wall of the temporal horn of the lateral ventricle.[57] It extends to the anterior margin of the ventricle, bringing it into the surgical field of many temporal epilepsy surgeries. Reports place the incidence of visual field defects up to 100% in ATL.[58] Selective procedures should theoretically limit damage to these structures and reduce the incidence of postoperative disturbances, but Egan and colleagues[58] found no difference in the incidence of visual field defects between middle temporal gyrus TC SAHC and modified ATL sparing the superior temporal gyrus. Mengesha and colleagues[59] found a similar frequency of visual field defects, but those in SAHC were less severe. Renowden and colleagues[60] demonstrated MRI evidence of damage to temporal white matter after both TS SAHC and TC SAHC, with an accompanying 53% incidence of incomplete quadrantanopia. Yeni and colleagues[61] found field defects on perimetric measurement in 36% of patients after TS SAHC, which was thought to be related to disruption of the Meyer loop during incision of the temporal stem. Lower incidence has been reported after subtemporal approaches.[9,47]

EVALUATION OF OUTCOME AND LONG-TERM RECOMMENDATIONS
Seizure Control

Control of seizures is the primary measure of success after SAHC. Two prospective randomized clinical trials have demonstrated the superiority of surgical treatment of MTLE over medical management, with 58% to 73% of surgical patients achieving seizure freedom versus 0% to 8% in the medical group.[3,4] An analysis by Jobst and Cascino[52] of 9 systematic reviews and 2 large case studies identified rates of seizure freedom following temporal lobe surgery of 34% to 73% (median 62.4%). However, no randomized clinical trials comparing SAHC with medical management alone have been performed to date. Therefore, rates of seizure control after SAHC are frequently compared with those following ATL.

Reported outcomes vary considerably, with most large series reporting that 50% to 90% of patients with MTLE are seizure free 1 year after SAHC.[11,16,26,52,62–70] For example, Mackenzie and colleagues[64] reported only 21% seizure freedom at 1 year after SAHC, whereas Tanriverdi and Olivier[68] reported 100% seizure freedom at the same interval. Several factors contribute to the variability of reported outcomes. First, although outcomes are frequently reported using the scale proposed by Engel and colleagues,[71] there is no clear consensus of what constitutes a satisfactory outcome. Second, MTLE is the common pathologic expression of a highly heterogeneous group of patients. Third, the technique, approach, and experience of the surgeon vary. Most importantly, accuracy of seizure localization and patient selection can vary independently from the technical success of surgery and exerts perhaps the highest influence on outcome.

There is evidence that seizures recur in patients who are initially seizure free.[16,62,72,73] Conversely, some studies suggest the effect of surgery is more durable. Wasade and colleagues[74] reported long-term outcomes of 253 patients up to 15 years after surgery, with a mean just more than 10 years. Among patients who had undergone temporal resection, 78% reported favorable (Engel class I and II) outcomes after more than 15 years.

Neuropsychological Outcomes

Although seizure control following surgery is of utmost concern, preservation of function is equally important. There is a paucity of high-quality data specific to SAHC,[52] and comparison is often made to the better-characterized risks following ATL (**Table 3**). Converging lines of evidence suggest that selective procedures have a superior functional outcome.[75,76]

A single controlled trial[77] comparing the memory outcomes of surgically and medically treated patients with temporal lobe epilepsy revealed that both groups had cognitive decline after 10 years, although seizure-free patients showed significant recovery of nonmemory function after surgery. Evidence from structured reviews and meta-analyses[78–82] suggests that intelligence is not affected by temporal lobe surgery. Verbal decline is the most common adverse event following temporal lobe resection, with 44% of patients with left-sided surgery and 20% with right-sided surgery showing a decline in verbal memory.[80] Nondominant resections do not seem to be associated with substantial nonverbal memory decline.[79,82] Naming deficits were present in 34% of dominant temporal lobe resections.[78,80] Evidence is accumulating that postoperative memory preservation after ATL depends on reorganization within the ipsilateral temporal lobe, including the posterior hippocampus, anterior cingulum, orbitofrontal cortex, and insula.[83]

Comparison of Anterior Temporal Lobectomy and Selective Amygdalohippocampectomy

Although selective procedures were developed in an effort to preserve function, no prospective, randomized controlled trials demonstrate superiority of SAHC or ATL. Two meta-analyses have supported a moderate advantage to seizure control with ATL for a 5% to 8% greater likelihood of seizure freedom.[84,85] A comparison study at 2 separate centers also suggested that ATL was slightly more effective in seizure control than SAHC, but the difference did not reach statistical significance.[86] However, SAHC led to significantly better results in visual encoding, verbal and short-term memory, and visual working memory. Many retrospective studies are available (see **Table 3**). Most studies suggest that, in appropriately selected patients, seizure control after surgery is similar for SAHC or ATL,[51,68,86–90] whereas others suggest ATL provides superior seizure control.[26,66]

There is evidence to suggest that neuropsychological outcomes are improved after selective procedures,[49,88,91–93] although some investigators found no significant differences.[94,95] Helmstaedter and colleagues[91] performed a detailed prospective study suggesting that, in surgery on the dominant side, ATL was less impactful on measures of verbal learning than SAHC, whereas on the nondominant side, selective surgery was less impactful. Interestingly, a study of category-related naming and object recognition found no

Table 3
Select publications comparing temporal lobe resection surgeries

Author, Year	Comparing	Study Design	Number of Patients	Duration of Follow-up (mo)	Classification of Favorable Outcome	Seizure Outcome	Cognitive Outcome
Helmstaedter et al,[65] 1996	ATL vs TS SAHC vs lesionectomy	Retro	59	3	Seizure free	No difference	Favors ALT
Mackenzie et al,[64] 1997	ATL vs SAHC	Retro	100	12	Engel III or better	Favors ATL	No difference
Clusmann et al,[87] 2002	ATL vs TS SAHC vs lesionectomy	Retro	321	38	Engel II or better	No difference	Favors SAHC
Clusmann et al,[26] 2004	ATL vs TS SAHC	Retro	89 (peds)	46	Engel II or better	Favors ATL	No difference on right, favors ATL on left
Hader et al,[109] 2005	ATL vs TC SAHC	Retro	72	Not specified	Engel II or better	No difference	No difference
Paglioli et al,[88] 2006	ATL vs TC SAHC	Pro	161	70	Engel I	No difference	Favors SAHC
Morino et al,[49] 2006	ATL vs TS SAHC	Retro	49	12	Seizure free	No difference	Favors SAHC
Bate et al,[66] 2007	CAH vs SAHC	Retro	114	12	Engel II or better	Favors ATL	Not reported
Tanriverdi and Olivier[68] 2007	CAH vs TC SAHC	Retro	72	12	Engel II or better	No difference	No difference
Helmstaedter et al,[91] 2008	Modified ATL vs TS SAHC	Pro	97	12	Only Engel I included	Only Engel I included	ATL better verbal learning, SAHC better figural learning
Tanriverdi et al,[62] 2008	CAH vs TC SAHC	Retro	100	60	Engel II or better	No difference	Not examined
Tanriverdi et al,[89] 2010	CAH vs TC SAHC	Retro	256	12	Engel II or better	No difference	No difference
Sagher et al,[86] 2012	ATL vs TC SAHC	Retro	96	44	Engel I	No difference	No difference
Bujarski et al,[72] 2013	ATL vs TC SAHC	Retro	69	81	Engel II or better	No difference	No difference
Wendling et al,[90] 2013	ATL vs TS SAHC	Retro	95	102	Seizure free	No difference	Favors SAHC
Mansouri et al,[110] 2014	ATL vs TC SAHC	Retro	54	40	Seizure free	No difference	No difference

Abbreviations: ATL, anterior temporal lobectomy; CAH, corticoamygdalohippocampectomy; peds, pediatric patients; Pro, prospective; Retro, retrospective; SAHC, selective amygdalohippocampectomy; TC SAHC, transcortical SAHC; TS SAHC, transsylvian SAHC.
Data from Refs.[26,49,62,64–66,72,86–91,109,110]

differences in patients undergoing ATL or selective procedures but superior outcomes following SAHC using laser interstitial thermal ablation.[96]

Although psychiatric outcomes are infrequently reported, Bujarski and colleagues[72] found no difference in depression or anxiety between ATL and SAHC. However, measures of paranoia increased overall with ATL and decreased overall with selective surgery. Taking this evidence together, SAHC seems to be as effective as ALT in patients with disease limited to the mesial temporal structures. Although not conclusive, the converging evidence suggests that selective resection likely offers better neurocognitive outcomes. More esoteric functions attributed to the anterolateral temporal lobe, such as semantic memory and relating conceptual understanding to social norms, are difficult to assess with standard neuropsychiatric paradigms but would theoretically be preserved by SAHC and be impaired after ATL.[97]

Comparison of Approaches to Selective Amygdalohippocampectomy

Data supporting the use of a particular surgical approach for SAHC are even more limited than data comparing SAHC with ATL. Lutz and colleagues[98] published a rare, prospective randomized trial comparing transsylvian and transcortical approaches. With the exception of phonemic fluency, which improved after transcortical procedures, there was no difference in seizure or

neuropsychological outcomes among the 80 patients studied. Other investigators have reported similar equality of seizure control between the two methods.[70,99] Inconsistency in testing techniques between studies, particularly in regard to neuropsychological function, make high-quality comparisons difficult, if not impossible (Table 4).

Von Rhein and colleagues[100] evaluated neuropsychological outcomes in matched cohorts of patients who underwent transsylvian and subtemporal approaches. Although the study design did not allow a comparison of seizure control, the investigators found more decline in verbal recognition memory in left TS SAHC and more decline in figural memory and verbal fluency with ST SAHC.

Very positive outcomes were reported in several studies of subtemporal approaches.[9,41,101–103] Takaya and colleagues[41] demonstrated postoperative improvement in glucose metabolism, verbal memory, attention, and delayed recall following a subtemporal approach in a limited number of patients without a control group. In a detailed analysis of 47 patients, Hill and colleagues[104] demonstrated decline in memory, verbal intellect, and naming in 29% to 38% of patients undergoing dominant hemisphere surgery, and declines in memory in 36% of patients undergoing nondominant hemisphere surgery using the minimal access approach described by the senior author. Current investigations are under way to determine if preoperative factors, such as hippocampal volume on MRI, can identify patients at higher risk for developing deficits after ST SAHC. Some

Table 4
Select publications comparing approaches to SAHC

Author, Year	Comparing	Study Design	Number of Patients	Duration of Follow-up (mo)	Seizure Outcome	Cognitive Outcome
Renowden et al,[60] 1995	TC SAHC vs TS SAHC	Retrospective	17	24	No difference	No difference
Lutz et al,[98] 2004	TC SAHC vs TS SAHC	Randomized prospective	80	7	No difference	Slightly better phonemic fluency in TC SAHC
von Rhein et al,[100] 2011	ST SAHC vs TS SAHC	Prospective cohort	26	12	Could not report	No difference
Drane et al,[96] 2015	TC SAHC vs ATL vs SLAHC	Nonrandomized prospective	58	6	No difference	Favored SLAHC in naming and recognition of famous faces

Abbreviation: SAHC, selective amygdalohippocampectomy; SLAHC, stereotactic laser amygdalohippocampectomy; ST SAHC, subtemporal SAHC; TC SAHC, transcortical SAHC; TS SAHC, transsylvian SAHC.
Data from Refs.[60,96,98,100]

surgeons,[98,105] in an effort to preserve cognitive function, have begun to explore other ablation techniques, such as laser thermal ablation. Early reports of these techniques suggest positive results with respect to preservation of function but with likely diminished long-term seizure control compared with complete mesial resections. Clinical trials comparing laser ablation with SAHC have been initiated to accurately quantify the potential disparity.

Long-term Follow-up

The authors advocate follow-up of patients who have undergone SAHC for at least 1 year after surgery. Because neuropsychological outcomes are central to evaluating the success of surgery, formal neuropsychological testing should be performed between 6 months and 1 year after surgery.

Discontinuation of Medical Treatment

If patients are seizure free after surgery, reducing or eliminating the use of antiepileptic drugs is possible. Reported rates of recurrent seizures with discontinuation of medical therapy vary, and little information is available for selective procedures alone. In reviews including ATL, 25% of MTLE surgery had seizures after stopping medical management, as opposed to 46% in neocortical epilepsy. Approximately 88% of those individuals who underwent temporal lobe procedures regained seizure freedom after reinitiating medications.[16] The authors' practice is to continue antiepileptic drugs at presurgical doses for 1 year after surgery, at which time a taper of medications may be initiated.

SUMMARY

SAHC has been developed in an attempt to treat MTLE while sparing temporal lobe structures sacrificed during ATL. The preponderance of the data suggests that SAHC is as effective in seizure control as ATL in appropriately selected patients. Although not conclusive, evidence suggests better preservation of neuropsychological function with SAHC.

A variety of approaches exist, each with theoretical advantages and disadvantages; but a review of the published data does not establish the superiority of a particular surgery. Each approach can be technically challenging. Certainly, the risk of deficits not related to resection of mesial temporal structures is present for all approaches. TS SAHC has a higher risk of vascular injury and stroke. TC SAHC is likely the easiest approach technically but does not spare the optic radiations, and it

results in the partial disconnection or injury to the spared lateral cortex. ST SAHC is the authors' favored approach because of the minimal access needed and because of the theoretical lack of disconnection or damage from the approach itself, although admittedly ventral visual pathway injury may contribute to memory decline beyond what would occur from hippocampectomy alone. Experience and skill on the part of the treating surgeon are necessities for the safe and efficacious execution of all the discussed approaches. Specialized training in a high-volume center is strongly recommended before attempting these techniques independently.

REFERENCES

1. Georgiadis I, Kapsalaki EZ, Fountas KN. Temporal lobe resective surgery for medically intractable epilepsy: a review of complications and side effects. Epilepsy Res Treat 2013;2013:752195.
2. Kovanda TJ, Tubbs RS, Cohen-Gadol AA. Transsylvian selective amygdalohippocampectomy for treatment of medial temporal lobe epilepsy: surgical technique and operative nuances to avoid complications. Surg Neurol Int 2014;5:133.
3. Wiebe S, Blume WT, Girvin JP, et al. A randomized, controlled trial of surgery for temporal-lobe epilepsy. N Engl J Med 2001;345(5):311–8.
4. Engel J Jr, McDermott MP, Wiebe S, et al. Early surgical therapy for drug-resistant temporal lobe epilepsy: a randomized trial. JAMA 2012;307(9):922–30.
5. Engel J Jr, Wiebe S, French J, et al. Practice parameter: temporal lobe and localized neocortical resections for epilepsy: report of the Quality Standards Subcommittee of the American Academy of Neurology, in association with the American Epilepsy Society and the American Association of Neurological Surgeons. Neurology 2003;60(4):538–47.
6. Widjaja E, Li B, Schinkel CD, et al. Cost-effectiveness of pediatric epilepsy surgery compared to medical treatment in children with intractable epilepsy. Epilepsy Res 2011;94(1–2):61–8.
7. Silfvenius H. Cost and cost-effectiveness of epilepsy surgery. Epilepsia 1999;40(Suppl 8):32–9.
8. Langfitt JT, Holloway RG, McDermott MP, et al. Health care costs decline after successful epilepsy surgery. Neurology 2007;68(16):1290–8.
9. Little AS, Smith KA, Kirlin K, et al. Modifications to the subtemporal selective amygdalohippocampectomy using a minimal-access technique: seizure and neuropsychological outcomes. J Neurosurg 2009;111(6):1263–74.
10. Yaşargil MG, Türe U, Boop FA. Selective amygdalohippocampectomy. In: Kaye AH, Black PM, editors.

Operative neurosurgery, vol. 2. London: Harcourt Publishers Limited; 2000. p. 1275–83.

11. Yaşargil MG, Krayenbuhl N, Roth P, et al. The selective amygdalohippocampectomy for intractable temporal limbic seizures. J Neurosurg 2010; 112(1):168–85.

12. Devinsky O. The myth of silent cortex and the morbidity of epileptogenic tissue: implications for temporal lobectomy. Epilepsy Behav 2005;7(3): 383–9.

13. Wheatley BM. Selective amygdalohippocampectomy: the trans-middle temporal gyrus approach. Neurosurg Focus 2008;25(3):E4.

14. Berg AT, Langfitt J, Shinnar S, et al. How long does it take for partial epilepsy to become intractable? Neurology 2003;60(2):186–90.

15. Kwan P, Arzimanoglou A, Berg AT, et al. Definition of drug resistant epilepsy: consensus proposal by the ad hoc Task Force of the ILAE Commission on Therapeutic Strategies. Epilepsia 2010;51(6): 1069–77.

16. Ryvlin P, Cross JH, Rheims S. Epilepsy surgery in children and adults. Lancet Neurol 2014;13(11): 1114–26.

17. French JA, Williamson PD, Thadani VM, et al. Characteristics of medial temporal lobe epilepsy: I. Results of history and physical examination. Ann Neurol 1993;34(6):774–80.

18. Radhakrishnan K, So EL, Silbert PL, et al. Predictors of outcome of anterior temporal lobectomy for intractable epilepsy: a multivariate study. Neurology 1998;51(2):465–71.

19. Cross JH, Jayakar P, Nordli D, et al. Proposed criteria for referral and evaluation of children for epilepsy surgery: recommendations of the Subcommission for Pediatric Epilepsy Surgery. Epilepsia 2006;47(6):952–9.

20. Spencer D, Burchiel K. Selective amygdalohippocampectomy. Epilepsy Res Treat 2012;2012: 382095 [Epub June 20, 2011].

21. Burch J, Hinde S, Palmer S. The clinical effectiveness and cost-effectiveness of technologies used to visualise the seizure focus in people with refractory epilepsy being considered for surgery: a systematic review and decision-analytical model. Health Technol Assess 2012;16:1–157.

22. Gil-Nagel A, Risinger MW. Ictal semiology in hippocampal versus extrahippocampal temporal lobe epilepsy. Brain 1997;120(Pt 1):183–92.

23. Kaiboriboon K, Nagarajan S, Mantle M, et al. Interictal MEG/MSI in intractable mesial temporal lobe epilepsy: spike yield and characterization. Clin Neurophysiol 2010;121(3):325–31.

24. Choi H, Carlino R, Heiman G, et al. Evaluation of duration of epilepsy prior to temporal lobe epilepsy surgery during the past two decades. Epilepsy Res 2009;86(2–3):224–7.

25. Haneef Z, Stern J, Dewar S, et al. Referral pattern for epilepsy surgery after evidence-based recommendations: a retrospective study. Neurology 2010;75(8):699–704.

26. Clusmann H, Kral T, Gleissner U, et al. Analysis of different types of resection for pediatric patients with temporal lobe epilepsy. Neurosurgery 2004; 54(4):847–59 [discussion: 859–60].

27. Datta A, Sinclair DB, Wheatley M, et al. Selective amygdalohippocampectomy: surgical outcome in children versus adults. Can J Neurol Sci 2009; 36(2):187–91.

28. Vajkoczy P, Krakow K, Stodieck S, et al. Modified approach for the selective treatment of temporal lobe epilepsy: transsylvian-transcisternal mesial en bloc resection. J Neurosurg 1998; 88(5):855–62.

29. Figueiredo EG, Deshmukh P, Nakaji P, et al. Anterior selective amygdalohippocampectomy: technical description and microsurgical anatomy. Neurosurgery 2010;66(3 Suppl Operative):45–53.

30. Chen HI, Bohman LE, Loevner LA, et al. Transorbital endoscopic amygdalohippocampectomy: a feasibility investigation. J Neurosurg 2014;120(6): 1428–36.

31. Türe U, Harput MV, Kaya AH, et al. The paramedian supracerebellar-transtentorial approach to the entire length of the mediobasal temporal region: an anatomical and clinical study. Laboratory investigation. J Neurosurg 2012;116(4):773–91.

32. Lafazanos S, Türe U, Harput MV, et al. Evaluating the importance of the tentorial angle in the paramedian supracerebellar-transtentorial approach for selective amygdalohippocampectomy. World Neurosurg 2015;83(5):836–41.

33. Shimizu H, Kawai K, Sunaga S, et al. Hippocampal transection for treatment of left temporal lobe epilepsy with preservation of verbal memory. J Clin Neurosci 2006;13(3):322–8.

34. Miyamoto S, Kataoka H, Ikeda A, et al. A combined subtemporal and transventricular/transchoroidal fissure approach to medial temporal lesions. Neurosurgery 2004;54(5):1162–7 [discussion: 1167–9].

35. Niemeyer P, Bello H. Amygdalohippocampectomy in temporal lobe epilepsy: microsurgical technique. Excerpta Med 1973;293:20.

36. Olivier A. Temporal resections in the surgical treatment of epilepsy. Epilepsy Res Suppl 1992;5:175–88.

37. Olivier A. Transcortical selective amygdalohippocampectomy in temporal lobe epilepsy. Can J Neurol Sci 2000;27(Suppl 1):S68–76 [discussion: S92–6].

38. Miyagi Y, Shima F, Ishido K, et al. Inferior temporal sulcus approach for amygdalohippocampectomy guided by a laser beam of stereotactic navigator. Neurosurgery 2003;52(5):1117–23 [discussion: 1123–4].

39. Yaşargil MG, Teddy PJ, Roth P. Selective amygdalo-hippocampectomy. Operative anatomy and surgical technique. Adv Tech Stand Neurosurg 1985;12:93–123.
40. Park TS, Bourgeois BF, Silbergeld DL, et al. Subtemporal transparahippocampal amygdalohippocampectomy for surgical treatment of mesial temporal lobe epilepsy. Technical note. J Neurosurg 1996; 85(6):1172–6.
41. Takaya S, Mikuni N, Mitsueda T, et al. Improved cerebral function in mesial temporal lobe epilepsy after subtemporal amygdalohippocampectomy. Brain 2009;132(Pt 1):185–94.
42. Hori T, Tabuchi S, Kurosaki M, et al. Subtemporal amygdalohippocampectomy for treating medically intractable temporal lobe epilepsy. Neurosurgery 1993;33(1):50–6 [discussion: 56–7].
43. Niemeyer P. The transventricular amygdala-hippocampectomy in the temporal lobe epilepsy. Temporal lobe epilepsy. Springfield (IL): Charles C. Thomas; 1958. p. 461–82.
44. Olivier A. Relevance of removal of limbic structures in surgery for temporal lobe epilepsy. Can J Neurol Sci 1991;18(4 Suppl):628–35.
45. Boling W. Minimal access keyhole surgery for mesial temporal lobe epilepsy. J Clin Neurosci 2010;17(9):1180–4.
46. Binder DK, Schramm J. Resective surgical techniques: mesial temporal lobe epilepsy. In: Luders HO, editor. Textbook of epilepsy surgery. London: Informa; 2008. p. 1083–92.
47. Thudium MO, Campos AR, Urbach H, et al. The basal temporal approach for mesial temporal surgery: sparing the Meyer loop with navigated diffusion tensor tractography. Neurosurgery 2010;67(2 Suppl Operative):385–90.
48. Wieser HG, Yaşargil MG. Selective amygdalohippocampectomy as a surgical treatment of mesiobasal limbic epilepsy. Surg Neurol 1982;17:445–57.
49. Morino M, Uda T, Naito K, et al. Comparison of neuropsychological outcomes after selective amygdalohippocampectomy versus anterior temporal lobectomy. Epilepsy Behav 2006;9(1):95–100.
50. Bahuleyan B, Fisher W, Robinson S, et al. Endoscopic transventricular selective amygdalohippocampectomy: cadaveric demonstration of a new operative approach. World Neurosurg 2013;80(1–2):178–82.
51. Sindou M, Guenot M, Isnard J, et al. Temporomesial epilepsy surgery: outcome and complications in 100 consecutive adult patients. Acta Neurochir (Wien) 2006;148(1):39–45.
52. Jobst BC, Cascino GD. Resective epilepsy surgery for drug-resistant focal epilepsy: a review. JAMA 2015;313(3):285–93.
53. McClelland S 3rd, Guo H, Okuyemi KS. Population-based analysis of morbidity and mortality following surgery for intractable temporal lobe epilepsy in the United States. Arch Neurol 2011;68(6):725–9.
54. Schaller C, Zentner J. Vasospastic reactions in response to the transsylvian approach. Surg Neurol 1998;49(2):170–5.
55. Schaller C, Jung A, Clusmann H, et al. Rate of vasospasm following the transsylvian versus transcortical approach for selective amygdalohippocampectomy. Neurol Res 2004;26(6):666–70.
56. Martens T, Merkel M, Holst B, et al. Vascular events after transsylvian selective amygdalohippocampectomy and impact on epilepsy outcome. Epilepsia 2014;55(5):763–9.
57. Kucukyuruk B, Richardson RM, Wen HT, et al. Microsurgical anatomy of the temporal lobe and its implications on temporal lobe epilepsy surgery. Epilepsy Res Treat 2012;2012:769825.
58. Egan RA, Shults WT, So N, et al. Visual field deficits in conventional anterior temporal lobectomy versus amygdalohippocampectomy. Neurology 2000; 55(12):1818–22.
59. Mengesha T, Abu-Ata M, Haas KF, et al. Visual field defects after selective amygdalohippocampectomy and standard temporal lobectomy. J Neuroophthalmol 2009;29(3):208–13.
60. Renowden SA, Matkovic Z, Adams CB, et al. Selective amygdalohippocampectomy for hippocampal sclerosis: postoperative MR appearance. AJNR Am J Neuroradiol 1995;16(9):1855–61.
61. Yeni SN, Tanriover N, Uyanik O, et al. Visual field defects in selective amygdalohippocampectomy for hippocampal sclerosis: the fate of Meyer's loop during the transsylvian approach to the temporal horn. Neurosurgery 2008;63(3):507–13 [discussion: 513–5].
62. Tanriverdi T, Olivier A, Poulin N, et al. Long-term seizure outcome after mesial temporal lobe epilepsy surgery: corticalamygdalohippocampectomy versus selective amygdalohippocampectomy. J Neurosurg 2008;108(3):517–24.
63. Spencer S, Huh L. Outcomes of epilepsy surgery in adults and children. Lancet Neurol 2008;7(6):525–37.
64. Mackenzie RA, Matheson J, Ellis M, et al. Selective versus non-selective temporal lobe surgery for epilepsy. J Clin Neurosci 1997;4(2):152–4.
65. Helmstaedter C, Elger CE, Hufnagel A, et al. Different effects of left anterior temporal lobectomy, selective amygdalohippocampectomy, temporal cortical lesionectomy on verbal learning, memory, and recognition. J Epilepsy 1996;9:39–45.
66. Bate H, Eldridge P, Varma T, et al. The seizure outcome after amygdalohippocampectomy and temporal lobectomy. Eur J Neurol 2007;14(1):90–4.
67. McIntosh AM, Wilson SJ, Berkovic SF. Seizure outcome after temporal lobectomy: current research practice and findings. Epilepsia 2001; 42(10):1288–307.

68. Tanriverdi T, Olivier A. Cognitive changes after uni-lateral cortico-amygdalohippocampectomy unilateral selective-amygdalohippocampectomy mesial temporal lobe epilepsy. Turk Neurosurg 2007;17(2):91–9.

69. Yaşargil MG, Wieser HG, Valavanis A, et al. Surgery and results of selective amygdala-hippocampectomy in one hundred patients with nonlesional limbic epilepsy. Neurosurg Clin N Am 1993;4(2):243–61.

70. Wieser HG, Ortega M, Friedman A, et al. Long-term seizure outcomes following amygdalohippocampectomy. J Neurosurg 2003;98(4):751–63.

71. Engel JJ, Van Ness P, Rasmussen TB, et al. Outcome with respect to epileptic seizures. In: Engel JJ, editor. Surgical treatment of the epilepsies. New York: Raven Press; 1993. p. 609–21.

72. Bujarski KA, Hirashima F, Roberts DW, et al. Long-term seizure, cognitive, and psychiatric outcome following trans-middle temporal gyrus amygdalohippocampectomy and standard temporal lobectomy. J Neurosurg 2013;119(1):16–23.

73. de Tisi J, Bell GS, Peacock JL, et al. The long-term outcome of adult epilepsy surgery, patterns of seizure remission, and relapse: a cohort study. Lancet 2011;378(9800):1388–95.

74. Wasade VS, Elisevich K, Tahir R, et al. Long-term seizure and psychosocial outcomes after resective surgery for intractable epilepsy. Epilepsy Behav 2015;43:122–7.

75. Schramm J. Temporal lobe epilepsy surgery and the quest for optimal extent of resection: a review. Epilepsia 2008;49(8):1296–307.

76. Helmstaedter C. Cognitive outcomes of different surgical approaches in temporal lobe epilepsy. Epileptic Disord 2013;15(3):221–39.

77. Helmstaedter C, Kurthen M, Lux S, et al. Chronic epilepsy and cognition: a longitudinal study in temporal lobe epilepsy. Ann Neurol 2003;54(4):425–32.

78. Ives-Deliperi VL, Butler JT. Naming outcomes of anterior temporal lobectomy in epilepsy patients: a systematic review of the literature. Epilepsy Behav 2012;24(2):194–8.

79. Lee TM, Yip JT, Jones-Gotman M. Memory deficits after resection from left or right anterior temporal lobe in humans: a meta-analytic review. Epilepsia 2002;43(3):283–91.

80. Sherman EM, Wiebe S, Fay-McClymont TB, et al. Neuropsychological outcomes after epilepsy surgery: systematic review and pooled estimates. Epilepsia 2011;52(5):857–69.

81. Téllez-Zenteno JF, Dhar R, Hernandez-Ronquillo L, et al. Long-term outcomes in epilepsy surgery: antiepileptic drugs, mortality, cognitive and psychosocial aspects. Brain 2007;130(Pt 2):334–45.

82. Vaz SA. Nonverbal memory functioning following right anterior temporal lobectomy: a meta-analytic review. Seizure 2004;13(7):446–52.

83. Duchowny M, Bhatia S. Epilepsy: preserving memory in temporal lobectomy-are networks the key? Nat Rev Neurol 2014;10(5):245–6.

84. Hu WH, Zhang C, Zhang K, et al. Selective amygdalohippocampectomy versus anterior temporal lobectomy in the management of mesial temporal lobe epilepsy: a meta-analysis of comparative studies. J Neurosurg 2013;119(5):1089–97.

85. Josephson CB, Dykeman J, Fiest KM, et al. Systematic review and meta-analysis of standard vs selective temporal lobe epilepsy surgery. Neurology 2013;80(18):1669–76.

86. Sagher O, Thawani JP, Etame AB, et al. Seizure outcomes and mesial resection volumes following selective amygdalohippocampectomy and temporal lobectomy. Neurosurg Focus 2012;32(3):E8.

87. Clusmann H, Schramm J, Kral T, et al. Prognostic factors and outcome after different types of resection for temporal lobe epilepsy. J Neurosurg 2002;97(5):1131–41.

88. Paglioli E, Palmini A, Portuguez M, et al. Seizure and memory outcome following temporal lobe surgery: selective compared with nonselective approaches for hippocampal sclerosis. J Neurosurg 2006;104(1):70–8.

89. Tanriverdi T, Dudley RW, Hasan A, et al. Memory outcome after temporal lobe epilepsy surgery: corticoamygdalohippocampectomy versus selective amygdalohippocampectomy. J Neurosurg 2010;113(6):1164–75.

90. Wendling AS, Hirsch E, Wisniewski I, et al. Selective amygdalohippocampectomy versus standard temporal lobectomy in patients with mesial temporal lobe epilepsy and unilateral hippocampal sclerosis. Epilepsy Res 2013;104(1–2):94–104.

91. Helmstaedter C, Richter S, Roske S, et al. Differential effects of temporal pole resection with amygdalohippocampectomy versus selective amygdalohippocampectomy on material-specific memory in patients with mesial temporal lobe epilepsy. Epilepsia 2008;49(1):88–97.

92. Helmstaedter C, Grunwald T, Lehnertz K, et al. Differential involvement of left temporolateral and temporomesial structures in verbal declarative learning and memory: evidence from temporal lobe epilepsy. Brain Cogn 1997;35(1):110–31.

93. Wendling AS, Steinhoff BJ, Bodin F, et al. Selective amygdalohippocampectomy versus standard temporal lobectomy in patients with mesiotemporal lobe epilepsy and unilateral hippocampal sclerosis: post-operative facial emotion recognition abilities. Epilepsy Res 2015;111:26–32.

94. Jones-Gotman M, Zatorre RJ, Olivier A, et al. Learning and retention of words and designs following excision from medial or lateral temporal-lobe structures. Neuropsychologia 1997;35(7):963–73.

95. Wolf RL, Ivnik RJ, Hirschorn KA, et al. Neurocognitive efficiency following left temporal lobectomy: standard versus limited resection. J Neurosurg 1993;79(1):76–83.

96. Drane DL, Loring DW, Voets NL, et al. Better object recognition and naming outcome with MRI-guided stereotactic laser amygdalohippocampotomy for temporal lobe epilepsy. Epilepsia 2015;56(1):101–13.

97. Bonner MF, Price AR. Where is the anterior temporal lobe and what does it do? J Neurosci 2013; 33(10):4213–5.

98. Lutz MT, Clusmann H, Elger CE, et al. Neuropsychological outcome after selective amygdalohippocampectomy with transsylvian versus transcortical approach: a randomized prospective clinical trial of surgery for temporal lobe epilepsy. Epilepsia 2004;45(7):809–16.

99. Cendes F, Dubeau F, Olivier A, et al. Increased neocortical spiking and surgical outcome after selective amygdalo-hippocampectomy. Epilepsy Res 1993;16(3):195–206.

100. von Rhein B, Nelles M, Urbach H, et al. Neuropsychological outcome after selective amygdalohippocampectomy: subtemporal versus transsylvian approach. J Neurol Neurosurg Psychiatry 2012; 83(9):887–93.

101. Hori T, Yamane F, Ochiai T, et al. Selective subtemporal amygdalohippocampectomy for refractory temporal lobe epilepsy: operative and neuropsychological outcomes. J Neurosurg 2007;106(1): 134–41.

102. Hori T, Yamane F, Ochiai T, et al. Subtemporal amygdalohippocampectomy prevents verbal memory impairment in the language-dominant hemisphere. Stereotact Funct Neurosurg 2003;80(1–4): 18–21.

103. Mikuni N, Miyamoto S, Ikeda A, et al. Subtemporal hippocampectomy preserving the basal temporal language area for intractable mesial temporal lobe epilepsy: preliminary results. Epilepsia 2006; 47(8):1347–53.

104. Hill SW, Gale SD, Pearson C, et al. Neuropsychological outcome following minimal access subtemporal selective amygdalohippocampectomy. Seizure 2012;21(5):353–60.

105. Gross RE, Mahmoudi B, Riley JP. Less is more: novel less-invasive surgical techniques for mesial temporal lobe epilepsy that minimize cognitive impairment. Curr Opin Neurol 2015;28(2):182–91.

106. Oertel J, Gaab MR, Runge U, et al. Neuronavigation and complication rate in epilepsy surgery. Neurosurg Rev 2004;27(3):214–7.

107. Acar G, Acar F, Miller J, et al. Seizure outcome following transcortical selective amygdalohippocampectomy in mesial temporal lobe epilepsy. Stereotact Funct Neurosurg 2008;86(5):314–9.

108. Bandt SK, Werner N, Dines J, et al. Trans-middle temporal gyrus selective amygdalohippocampectomy for medically intractable mesial temporal lobe epilepsy in adults: seizure response rates, complications, and neuropsychological outcomes. Epilepsy Behav 2013;28(1):17–21.

109. Hader WJ, Pillay N, Myles ST, et al. The benefit of selective over standard surgical resections in the treatment of intractable temporal lobe epilepsy. Epilepsia 2005;46:253–60.

110. Mansouri A, Fallah A, McAndrews MP, et al. Neurocognitive and seizure outcomes of selective amygdalohippocampectomy versus anterior temporal lobectomy for mesial temporal lobe epilepsy. Epilepsy Res Treat 2014;2014:306382.

Hippocampal Transections for Epilepsy

Arun Angelo Patil, MD[a,*], Andrea Jennifer Chamczuk, MD, MSc[a], Richard V. Andrews, MD[b]

KEYWORDS

• Multiple hippocampal transection • Temporal lobe epilepsy • Long-term outcome • Verbal memory

KEY POINTS

• Multiple hippocampal transection (MHT), supplemented with multiple subpial transection (MST) and limited cortical resection, is a relatively safe procedure that affords excellent seizure control that is equal to or exceeds the results typically achieved with standard temporal lobectomy; in addition, verbal memory and stem cells are preserved.

• Intraoperative electrocorticography is of paramount importance in ensuring that all seizure foci are abolished. This is especially true for nonresective procedures like MST and MHT.

• This approach is best suited in patients who are not suitable candidates for standard temporal lobectomy due to failed Wada test, dominant temporal lobe epilepsy, or the absence of hippocampal sclerosis.

INTRODUCTION

Representing nearly 25% of all cases of epilepsy, of which an estimated 70% are referred for consideration of surgical intervention, temporal lobe epilepsy (TLE) represents the single most common type of seizure disorder.[1–3] Unfortunately, approximately 30% of patients with TLE fail to achieve satisfactory control of their seizures with antiepileptic medications. In addition, many of them suffer from side effects of antiepileptic drugs when an attempt is made to increase their dosage in order to reduce the frequency of seizures.[4–6] Surgical intervention offers these patients the possibility of seizure-freedom or near seizure-freedom with a reduced dependency on antiepileptic medication.[5]

Treatment of intractable TLE classically involves resection of the anterior part of the temporal lobe, including resection of the parahippocampal gyrus, amygdala, hippocampus, and the fimbria. This procedure is considered the gold standard in the treatment of TLE.[7] Resection of the hippocampus is performed because the hippocampus is involved in the generation and propagation of seizures, and there is a close association between hippocampal sclerosis and TLE.

However, resection of the hippocampus is undesirable because it is an integral part of the limbic system, has important connections with the entorhinal cortex, is the site for new memory formation, including auditory and visual organization, and is involved in memory retrieval. Furthermore, temporal lobe neocortex is essential for accurate perception and interpretation of social communication, recognizing familiar faces and facial emotions, interpreting voice, understanding a person's intentions and emotions from their body posture, gestures, and movements, and participation in precipitating emotional empathy.[8,9]

Therefore, complications of standard temporal lobectomy include impairment of social cognition, decline in verbal memory, general intelligence, emotional and vocational disturbances, psychosis, character disorders, depression, and linguistic dysfunctions.[9–19] Although the Wada test is

None of the authors have commercial interest related to this article; this is an original work of the authors.
[a] Creighton University Medical Center, Division of Neurosurgery, 601 North 30th Street, Omaha, NE 68131, USA; [b] 11930 Arbor Street, Omaha, NE 68144, USA
* Corresponding author.
E-mail address: arun.patil@alegent.org

routinely used to ascertain the dominant side for memory, Wada asymmetry (using mixed stimuli) fails to predict postoperative verbal memory.[12] Furthermore, there is a higher risk of memory dysfunction in those cases with minimal or no sclerosis, or those in whom the dominant hemisphere is involved.[14,15] Furthermore, the subventricular and subgranular zones of the hippocampus, which are the main source of neural progenitor cells,[20–23] are resected. These cells are critical in the ongoing repair process of the brain following trauma or ischemic injuries.[24–28]

In order to obviate the problems associated with temporal lobectomy and eliminate the need for brain tissue resection, several neuromodulator methods are presently under trial. They include deep brain stimulation, vagal nerve stimulation, and transcranial magnetic stimulation. Several targets in the brain, including the anterior thalamus, the centromedian nucleus of the thalamus, the subthalamic nucleus, and the hippocampus, have been used as targets for deep brain stimulation. Despite some encouraging initial results using these treatment modalities, their clinical value remains to be determined because none of them to date have produced results equal to anterior temporal lobectomy.[29] Other methods under investigation are selective stereotactic destruction of the hippocampus using radiofrequency current, ultrasound, LASER (light amplification by stimulated emission of radiation), and stereotactic radiation.[30] However, these methods do not address seizures originating from the extrahippocampal structures.[31–35] In addition, in these methods, neural stem cells within the hippocampus are destroyed.

Against this background, multiple hippocampal transection (MHT) is a procedure worth considering. MHT is a novel procedure[36–39] in which the longitudinal fibers responsible for seizure propagation are transected at several points along the length of the hippocampus (**Fig. 1**) without resecting the hippocampus. MHT preserves the hippocampus and the stem cells within it and decreases the probability of affecting the hippocampal functions. Furthermore, in order to disrupt seizure circuits in the extrahippocampal cortex, multiple subpial transection (MST) is performed. In addition, when MST fails to abolish epileptogenic activity, minimal cortical resection is performed.[39] In this article, the authors review this approach of treatment of intractable TLE.

PATIENT EVALUATION OVERVIEW

Patients presenting with treatment-refractory TLE typically have at least 1 to 3 seizures per week with many having more than one seizure per day. Routine preoperative evaluation includes video electroencephalography (EEG), magnetic resonance (MR) imaging, magnetoencephalography and PET scans, neuropsychological evaluation, Wada test, and EEG studies using depth and subdural electrodes. Patients are maintained off antiepileptic drugs (AED) 2 days before surgery. Anesthesia is induced using methohexital, and seizure-suppressing drugs (eg, benzodiazepine, propofol) are not used.

SURGICAL PROCEDURE

First, the temporal horn is opened through the middle temporal gyrus using the BrainLab Neuronavigation System (BrainLab AG, Feldkirchen, Germany). Subsequently, using the operative microscope, MHTs are performed at 4- to 5-mm intervals over the head, body, and proximal portions of the tail of the hippocampus. During the procedure, a small incision is made on the ventricular surface of the hippocampus through the alveus using a no. 11 blade scalpel (**Fig. 2**). The knife is inserted no more than a millimeter deep. Through this opening a blunt wire loop 3 or 5 mm in diameter is vertically inserted into the gray matter of the hippocampus to perform transection through the entire transverse diameter of the hippocampus. At the head and proximal part of the body of the hippocampus, the 5-mm-diameter loop is used. At the distal body and proximal tail, a 3-mm-diameter loop is used. The thickness of the hippocampus is measured on coronal MR images at different points, with the depth of insertion of the loop tailored to those distances. In addition, the resistance offered by the alveus on the other side is an indication to stop further insertion. The loop is also moved side to side inside the hippocampus within the limits of the alveus in order to ensure adequate transection within the alveus. The fimbria is left intact. Should the preoperative depth electrode recording show epileptogenic activity in the amygdala, it is excised through the temporal horn. Further details regarding this procedure have been described in previous publications.[37,39]

Next, MST is performed over the lateral and basal surfaces of the temporal lobe in and around areas that showed epileptogenic activity based on preoperative EEG studies. The area usually extends 5 to 7 cm posterior to the tip of the temporal lobe and includes the parahippocampal gyrus and the entorhinal cortex.

Following this, intraoperative electrocorticography (ECoG) is recorded for an hour with intracranial electrodes over the hippocampal and

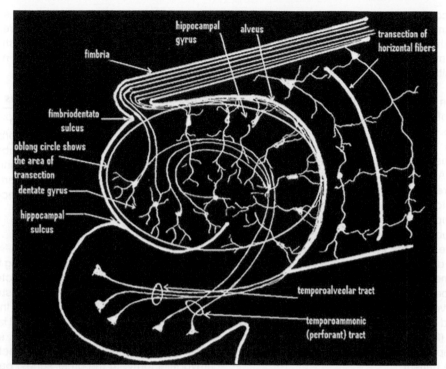

Fig. 1. Major tracts of the hippocampus in relation to transection. (*Data from* Patil AA, Andrews RV. Long term follow-up after multiple hippocampal transection (MHT). Seizure 2013; 22:731–4; and Shimizu H, Kawai K, Sunaga S, et al. Hippocampal transection for treatment of left temporal lobe epilepsy with preservation of memory. J Clin Neurosci 2006;13:322–8.)

neocortical surfaces with the patient on minimal anesthetic agents. If recordings show areas of persistent epileptogenic activity, transections are repeated over areas that showed such activity. Subsequently, another set of intraoperative ECoG is recorded. If persistent epileptogenic areas are noted, they are resected. Neither the hippocampus nor the entorhinal cortex is ever resected. Once again, the ECoG recording is repeated. If this shows epileptogenic activity, the resection is extended. This process is repeated as needed until the ECoG is free of all epileptogenic activity. In the authors' series,[39] the length of the resection

posterior to the temporal tip measured 1.5 to 2.5 cm.

EVALUATION OF OUTCOME AND LONG-TERM RECOMMENDATIONS

Neuropsychological tests before surgery and 3 to 6 months after surgery are obtained. These tests included the Wechsler intelligence score, Wechsler memory scale, repeatable battery for the assessment of neurologic state Form A, wide-range achievement test, trail making test, grooved pegboard task, controlled word association test,

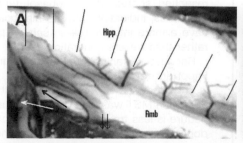
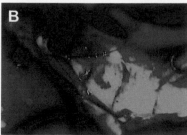

Fig. 2. (*A*) Anatomy of the temporal horn. Fimb, fimbria; Hipp, hippocampus. Single white arrow: amygdala; Double black arrow: choroid plexus; single black arrow: uncal recess. (*B*) Transverse cuts in the hippocampus.

Connor's continuous performance test, and the Boston naming test. The results from different tests are then scored and averaged for verbal and visual memory.

The results from both studies are summarized in **Table 1**.

In brief, in a series of 15 patients with a minimum follow-up of 2 years, Patil and Andrews[39] found that 94.7% of the patients were seizure free (Engel's class 1). Only one (5.3%) had rare seizures (Engel's class 2). Although all patients were maintained on AEDs, the number of required mediations was reduced from 3 to 4 (preoperatively) to 2 to 3 (postoperatively). Reduction of medications was accomplished based on postoperative follow-up EEG studies and the degree of seizure control. Most of the patients in this series had failed the Wada test during the preoperative evaluation.

Verbal memory was either improved or stable after the operation (77.8%/22.2%). Visual memory was improved or stable in most patients (44.4%/33.4%) and only slightly deteriorated in a minority of patients (22.2%). The sole neurologic complication of temporary word finding difficulty was present in one patient.

In their series of 21 patients, Shimizu and colleagues[36] likewise achieved excellent results, with an 82% seizure-free rate after the procedure. Twelve percent of patients improved in their clinical status with rare persistent seizures,

and 6% of patients were considered significantly improved. Verbal memory was preserved in 87.5%, and only one patient demonstrated transient decline in verbal memory at 1 month with subsequent resolution by 6 month.

Treatment Resistance/Complications

Patil and Andrews[39] had only one patient in their series that developed temporary word-finding difficulty, which resolved subsequently. Shimizu and colleagues[36] reported only one patient who had a decreased verbal memory score postprocedure that subsequently recovered at 6-month follow-up.

SUMMARY/DISCUSSION

There are many objections to resecting the hippocampus during anterior temporal lobectomy operation. Most of these have been listed in the introduction section of this article. In addition, based on outcome studies, results of 2 large series of patients were compared. In one series, the patients had anterior temporal lobectomy with amygdalectomy. In the other series, patients had hippocampectomy with amygdalectomy. The comparison showed that hippocampectomy did not add to the benefit.[40,41] Furthermore, despite the close association between TLE and hippocampal sclerosis,[42,43] and despite animal experimental studies that have identified CA3 as the site of origin of epileptic discharges,[44] some authors refute the concept of abnormal sclerotic hippocampus playing a role in seizure genesis[34] stating that other limbic areas and extrahippocampal structures, such as the entorhinal cortex, may be responsible for seizure generation.[34,35,45] Moreover, the interictal spike in the hippocampus may actually inhibit seizure onset, potentially explaining why seizures generated within the hippocampus fail to ever become generalized.[46] Siegel and colleagues[33] noted that even when selective amygdalohippocampectomy was performed for TLE, seizure control was correlated not only to the extent of hippocampal resection but also to the resection scores of mediobasal temporal lobe structures, indicating that the hippocampus may have a more integral role in seizure propagation rather than seizure generation itself.[44]

Because extrahippocampal structures play an important role in seizure generation, MHT alone is not adequate. Therefore, in the present approach MST was also done. Because this procedure is less traumatic than resection, it can be done over a large area, enabling treatment of areas that are usually not included in standard temporal lobectomy. MST, however, may not abolish all

Table 1
Results of 2 series

	Patil and Andrews,[39] 2013	Shimizu et al,[36] 2006
Length of follow-up (y)	2	1
N	15	21
Seizure outcome		
Seizure freedom	94.7%	82%
Rare seizure	5.3%	12%
Significantly improved	N/A	6%
Verbal memory		
Improved	77.8%	N/A
Preserved	22.2%	87.5%
Visual memory		
Improved	44.4%	N/A
Stable	33.3%	N/A
Slightly deteriorated	22.2%	N/A

seizure foci. In such cases, cortical resection is needed. However, because MST drastically reduces the epileptogenic areas, very small areas of cortical resection are needed. In the authors' series,[39] this area was always at the tip of the temporal lobe, indicating that MST may not be as effective at the temporal tip. The reason for this could be because it is extremely difficult to perform MST over the cortex in deep sulci at the temporal tip because of accessibility.

Organized perpendicular to the length of the hippocampus, most of the fiber tracts within the hippocampus are integral to hippocampal function. These circuits include perforant pathways from the entorhinal cortex to the dentate gyrus and CA3 area, Schaffer collateral pathway from CA3 to CA1, and from CA1 to the subiculum to the entorhinal cortex.[34] Conversely, tracts responsible for seizure propagation run longitudinally along the length of the hippocampus, and these include the longitudinal axonal projections of CA3 pyramidal cells, longitudinal fiber systems in the dentate gyrus, and longitudinal axonal ramifications in the inner and outer molecular layers. Moreover, signal propagation along these longitudinal tracts is in the anterior-posterior direction with a fixed peak-to-peak interval.[45] In addition, there is synchronization between different hippocampal regions and between the hippocampus and the ipsilateral anterior parahippocampal gyrus. Therefore, 1 or 2 transections between the head and body of the hippocampus can abolish hippocampal spikes that are synchronized along the entire axis of the hippocampus,[35] unlike MST, which disrupts only local synchrony.

Vertical cuts in the hippocampus afford disruption of the longitudinal fibers within the hippocampus without damaging the vertical fibers. Therefore, seizure propagation is disrupted without deleterious effect to hippocampal functions. The key to successful outcome is to transect the entire thickness of the hippocampal gray matter in a plane perpendicular to the length of the hippocampus and parallel to the hippocampal digitations, albeit without including the fimbria, which is the main outflow pathway of the hippocampus.

Patil and Andrews[39] used stereotactic navigation when entering the temporal horn in order to minimize collateral damage to the brain. The alveus, the outer covering of the hippocampus, is tough tissue that mandates the use of a sharp knife and a loop to gain entry into the gray matter. The latter was used to perform the transections, because the loop is blunt and thus unlikely to cut through the alveus on the other side and damage the critical neurovascular structures medial to the hippocampus.

Patil and Andrews[39] and Shimizu and colleagues[36] report seizure-free percentages of 94.7 and 82, respectively. These results are better than those reported for temporal lobectomy.[7] These results may be due to the fact that MST was performed in areas ordinarily not resected during standard temporal lobectomy. Preservation of verbal memory and minimal to no lasting neurologic complication are most probably a result of the tissue resection being minimal.

Resection of the neocortex by Patil's group was performed when intraoperative ECoG indicated that the seizure circuits in that area were refractory to MST. The areas of resection were very small as compared with the area that initially showed epileptogenic activity, indicating that although MST may not abolish epileptogenic activity in all areas, it does reduce the area with epileptogenic activity. The fact that all patients needed repeat MST and some patients needed minimal resection based on intraoperative ECoG underscores that one MST pass may be insufficient to abolish epileptogenic activity in all areas. It also emphasizes the importance of intraoperative ECoG recording during MST surgery. Furthermore, the fact that all patients needed repeat MST after MHT and MST indicates that MHT alone will not abolish seizure activity.

In summary, MHT coupled with MST, and when needed, minimal cortical resection, can abolish seizures in a very high percentage of patients with TLE. The risks with this procedure are minimal, and the chance of preserving verbal memory is high. Therefore, it is worthwhile to further evaluate this procedure as an alternative to temporal lobectomy, especially if a patient fails the Wada test or does not have significant sclerosis on the offending side, or if the offending side is the dominant hemisphere.

REFERENCES

1. Williamson PD, Engel J Jr. Complex partial seizures. In: Engel J Jr, Pedley TA, editors. Epilepsy: a comprehensive textbook. Philadelphia; New York: Lippincott-Raven; 1998. p. 557–66.

2. Zimmerman RS, Sirven JI. An overview of surgery for chronic seizures. Mayo Clin Proc 2003;78:109–17.

3. Kwong KL, Sung WY, Wong SN, et al. Early predictors of medical intractability in childhood epilepsy. Pediatr Neurol 2003;29:46–52.

4. Wiebe S, Blume WT, Girvin JP, et al. A randomized, controlled trial of surgery for temporal lobe epilepsy. N Engl J Med 2001;345:311–8.

5. Singhvi JP, Washney IM, Lal V, et al. Profile of intractable epilepsy in a tertiary referral center. Neurol India 2000;48:351–6.

6. McIntosh AM, Wilson SJ, Berkoic SF. Seizure outcome after temporal lobectomy: current research practice and findings. Epilepsia 2001;42:1288–307.

7. Doyle WK, Spencer DD. Anterior temporal lobe resections. In: Engel JJ, Pedley TA, editors. Epilepsy: a comprehensive textbook. Philadelphia: Lippincott-Raven Publishers; 1997. p. 1807–17.

8. Eichenbaum H, Yonelinas AP, Ranganath C. The medial temporal lobe and recognition memory. Annu Rev Neurosci 2007;30:123–52.

9. Squire LR. Memory and the hippocampus: a synthesis from findings with rats, monkeys, and humans. Psychol Rev 1992;99:195–231.

10. Alpherts WC, Vermeulen J, van Rijen PC, et al. Dutch collaborative epilepsy surgery programs: verbal memory decline after temporal lobe epilepsy surgery?: A 6-year multiple assessment follow-up study. Neurology 2006;67:626–31.

11. Bebrens B, Sehramm J, Zentner J, et al. Surgical and neurological complications in a series of 708 epilepsy surgery procedures. Neurosurgery 1997; 41:1–9.

12. Baxendale S, Thompson P, Harkness W, et al. The role of the intracarotid amobarbital procedure in predicting verbal decline after temporal lobe resection. Epilepsia 2007;48:546–52.

13. Glessner U, Helmstaedter C, Schramm J, et al. Memory outcome after seizure amydalohippocampectomy: a study in 140 patients with temporal lobe epilepsy. Epilepsia 2002;43:87–95.

14. Helmstaedter C. Neuropsychological aspects of epilepsy surgery. Epilepsy Behav 2004;5(Suppl): S45–50.

15. Herman B, Wyler A, Somes G, et al. Psychological status of the mesial temporal lobe predicts memory outcome from left anterior temporal lobectomy. Neurosurgery 1992;31:652–7.

16. LoGalbo A, Sawrie S, Roth DI, et al. Verbal memory outcome in patients with normal preoperative verbal memory and left mesial temporal sclerosis. Epilepsy Behav 2005;6:337–41.

17. Nunn JA, Graydon FJX, Polkey CE, et al. Differential spatial memory impairment after right temporal lobectomy demonstrated using temporal titration. Brain 1999;122:47–59.

18. Seidenberg M, Hermann B, Wyler AR, et al. Neuropsychological outcome following anterior temporal lobectomy in patients with and without the syndrome of mesial temporal lobe epilepsy. Neuropsychology 1998;12(2):303–16.

19. Stoup E, Langfitt J, Berg M, et al. Predicting verbal memory decline following anterior temporal lobectomy (ATL). Neurology 2003;60:1266–76.

20. Kaslin J, Ganz J, Brand M. Proliferation neurogenesis and regeneration in the adult non-mammalian vertebrae brain. Philos Trans R Soc Lond B Biol Sci 2007;363:101–22.

21. Ming GI, Song H. Adult neurogenesis in the mammalian central nervous system. Annu Rev Neurosci 2005;28:223–50.

22. Pencea V, Bingaman KD, Freedman LJ, et al. Neurogenesis in the subventricular zone and rostral migratory stream of the neonatal and adult primate forebrain. Exp Neurol 2001;172:1–16.

23. Riquelme PA, Drapeau E, Doetsch F. Brain microecologies: neural stem cell niches in the adult mammalian. Philos Trans R Soc Lond B Biol Sci 2007;363:123–37.

24. Gao X, Enikolopov G, Chen J. Moderate traumatic brain injury promotes proliferation of quiescent neural progenitors in adult hippocampus. Exp Neurol 2009;219:516–23.

25. Gould B, Tanapat P. Lesion-induced proliferation of neuronal progenitors in the dentate gyrus of the adult rat. Neuroscience 1997;80:427–36.

26. Jin K, Sun Y, Xie L, et al. Directed migration of neuronal precursors into the ischemic cerebral cortex and striatum. Mol Cell Neurosci 2003;24:171–89.

27. Leker RR. Fate and manipulations of endogenous stem cells following brain ischemia. Expert Opin Biol Ther 2009;9:1117–25.

28. Liu J, Solway K, Messing RO, et al. Increased neurogenesis in the dentate gyrus after transient global ischemia in gerbils. J Neurosci 1998;18: 7768–78.

29. Andrews RJ. Neuroprotection trek–the next generation: neuromodulation I. Techniques–deep brain stimulation, vagus nerve stimulation, and transcranial magnetic stimulation. Ann N Y Acad Sci 2003; 993:1–13.

30. Nowell M, Miserocchi A, McEvoy AW, et al. Advances in epilepsy surgery. J Neurol Neurosurg Psychiatry 2014;85(11):1273–9.

31. Avoli M, D'Antuono M, Louvel J, et al. Network and pharmacological mechanisms leading to epileptiform synchronization in the limbic system in vitro. Prog Neurobiol 2002;68:167–207.

32. Bartolomei F, Khalil M, Wendling F, et al. Entorhinal cortex involvement in human mesial temporal lobe epilepsy: an electrophysiologic and volumetric study. Epilepsia 2005;46:677–87.

33. Siegel AM, Wieser HG, Wichmann W, et al. Relationships between MR-imaged total amount of tissue removed, resection scores of specific mediobasal limbic subcompartments and clinical outcome following selective amygdalohippocampectomy. Epilepsy Res 1990;6(1):56–65.

34. Wennberg R, Arruda F, Quesney L, et al. Preeminence of extrahippocampal structures in the generation of mesial temporal seizures: evidence from human depth electrode recordings. Epilepsia 2002;43:716–26.

35. Amaral D, Lavenex P. Hippocampal neuroanatomy. In: Andersen P, Morris R, Amaral D, et al, editors.

The hippocampus book. Oxford (United Kingdom): Oxford University Press; 2006 [Chapter 3].

36. Shimizu H, Kawai K, Sunaga S, et al. Hippocampal transection for treatment of left temporal lobe epilepsy with preservation of memory. J Clin Neurosci 2006;13:322–8.

37. Patil AA, Andrews RA. Multiple hippocampal transections (MHT) – preliminary report. World Neurosurg 2010;74(6):645–9.

38. Sunaga S, Morino M, Kusakabe T, et al. Efficacy of hippocampal transection for left temporal lobe epilepsy without hippocampal atrophy. Epilepsy Behav 2011;21(1):94–9.

39. Patil AA, Andrews RV. Long term follow-up after multiple hippocampal transection (MHT). Seizure 2013; 22:731–4.

40. Rasmussen T, Feindel W. Temporal lobectomy: review of 100 cases with major hippocampectomy. Can J Neurol Sci 1991;18:601–2.

41. Feindel W, Rasmussen T. Temporal lobectomy with amygdalectomy and minimal hippocampal resection. Review of 100 cases. Can J Neurol Sci 1991;18:603–5.

42. Babb TL, Brown WJ. Pathological findings in epilepsy. In: Engel J Jr, editor. Surgical treatment of the epilepsies. New York: Raven Press; 1987. p. 511–40.

43. Swanson TH. The pathophysiology of human mesial temporal lobe epilepsy. J Clin Neurophysiol 1995;12: 2–22.

44. Barbarosie M, Avoli M. CA3-driven hippocampal–entorhinal loop controls rather than sustains in vitro limbic seizures. J Neurosci 1997;17:9308–14.

45. Umeoka SC, Lüders HO, Turnbull JP, et al. Requirement of longitudinal synchrony of epileptiform discharges in the hippocampus for seizure generation: a pilot study. J Neurosurg 2012;116:513–24.

46. Trevino M, Vivar C, Gutierrez R. Oscillatory activity in the CA3 hippocampal area is depressed by aberrant GABAergic transmission from the dentate gyrus after seizures. J Neurosci 2007;27:251–9.

History and Technical Approaches and Considerations for Ablative Surgery for Epilepsy

Saurabh Sinha, MD, Shabbar F. Danish, MD*

KEYWORDS

• Epilepsy • Ablative neurosurgery • Stereotactic neurosurgery • Electroencephalography • History

KEY POINTS

• From post-traumatic epilepsy to non–lesional epilepsy, the history of epilepsy surgery has proceeded through phases of refined methods of localization of macroscopic and microscopic pathology.
• Current forms of minimally invasive stereotactic procedures, increasing in popularity today, draw from important diagnostic and operative advances. As such, they should be understood in an historical context.
• The history of epilepsy surgery has demonstrated the importance of collaboration between neurology, neurosurgery, electrophysiology and more for optimal treatment of epilepsy.

INTRODUCTION

Although the idea of neurosurgical intervention to treat epilepsy dates back to antiquity with the practice of trephination,[1] advances in understanding brain function in the 1800s led to more precise localization. Refinements in localization of pathology characterize advances throughout the history of ablative epilepsy surgery. The late 1800s to early 1900s emphasized localization based on clinical symptoms. The advent of electroencephalography (EEG) in the mid-1900s allowed for the surgical treatment of nonlesional epilepsy while improving targeting of pathology, marking a new frontier for epilepsy surgery. The concurrent development of stereotaxy for neurosurgery allowed for increased precision of the surgical approach and motivates present-day advances in minimally invasive ablative epilepsy surgery.

This article discusses the major historical moments that defined the development and refinement of ablative epilepsy surgery, starting with

Victor Horsley's landmark case series in 1886 and discussing the evolution of the field over the next century (**Tables 1** and **2**). Because mesial temporal lobe epilepsy (MTLE) is the form of epilepsy for which neurosurgical intervention is most commonly used, the evolution of the surgical approach for MTLE is discussed as a representative example, but other forms of epilepsy are discussed when appropriate. How these advances have led to today's ablative epilepsy surgery is then discussed, historical context for ablative technology is provided, and current technical approaches discussed.

HISTORY

Sensorimotor Cortices and Early Localization

The modern era of ablative epilepsy surgery is often noted to have begun in 1886 with Horsley's report of surgical excision of tumors in 3 cases of focal Jacksonian epilepsy.[2] But important advancements in the understanding of brain function

Disclosures: S.F. Danish received an honorarium from Visualase Inc.
Department of Neurosurgery, Rutgers Robert Wood Johnson Medical School, 125 Paterson Street, New Brunswick, NJ 08901, USA
* Corresponding author. CAB Suite 2100, 125 Paterson Street, New Brunswick, NJ 08901.
E-mail address: shabbar.danish@rutgers.edu

Neurosurg Clin N Am 27 (2016) 27–36
http://dx.doi.org/10.1016/j.nec.2015.08.002
1042-3680/16/$ – see front matter © 2016 Elsevier Inc. All rights reserved.

Table 1
Important figures in the history of epilepsy surgery

Name(s)	Contribution	Relevant Article(s)
John Hughlings Jackson	Developed analytical approach to neurologic problems, defined Jacksonian march	Hughlings Jackson, 1869 York and Steinberg, 2011
Victor Horsley	Reported first craniotomies for posttraumatic epilepsy	Horsley, 1886
Fedor Krause	Championed epilepsy surgery, pushed for surgical treatment of nonlesional epilepsy	Krause and Schum, 1932
Wilder Penfield	Founded MNI, standardized ATL	Penfield and Baldwin, 1952
Herbert Jasper	Helped incorporate EEG with neurosurgery	Jasper, 1941
F.A. Gibbs, E.L. Gibbs, and W.G. Lennox	Classified abnormal EEG patterns	Gibbs et al, 1937
J. Talairach and J. Bancaud	Standardization of stereotactic approach, SEEG	Talairach et al, 1957 Mazoyer, 2008
Theodore Rasmussen	Histopathology of epilepsy and outcomes of epilepsy surgery, defined Rasmussen encephalitis	Stahnisch and Nakashima, 2013

preceded this development. The work of John Hughlings Jackson was crucial in providing the impetus for exploring the brain in epilepsy. In promoting a physical basis for neurologic pathology and shunning the appeal to metaphysics that characterized the understanding of the brain in the early 1800s, Hughlings Jackson brought the scientific method squarely into the arena of neurology.[3] This approach led to his characterization, in 1867, of the somatotopic procession of a seizure through the motor cortex that bears his name: the Jacksonian march.[4]

Table 2
Landmark case studies in the history of epilepsy surgery

Article	Description
Horsley, 1886	3 Patients with posttraumatic epilepsy undergoing craniotomies
Penfield and Flanigan, 1950	68 Patients with MTLE, some with uncus resection and hippocampectomies
Penfield and Baldwin, 1952	Standardization of ATL
Niemeyer and Bello, 1973	SelAH first described
Wiebe and colleagues, 2001	RCT demonstrating ATL as gold standard for treatment-refractory MTLE

Intrigued and influenced by his colleague's findings,[5] Horsley, operating in England, proceeded with craniotomies to treat epilepsy, as recorded in the aforementioned case series.[6] In this case series, the first of its kind, Horsley documented 3 cases in which he combined analysis of clinical presentation with cortical stimulation to localize a precise region for excision. The first patient, originally a patient of Hughlings Jackson, was a 22 year old with posttraumatic epilepsy caused by a skull fracture at age 15.[7] The patient did well, as did the 2 others reported in the series.[6] From the success of these procedures emerged an important pattern: using clinical presentation for surgical planning. This trend crystallized distinctly in 1909, a "landmark year for epilepsy."[5] Among other important events in the year, such as Horsley giving a major lecture about his cases, the International League Against Epilepsy had its first meeting, and the surgical treatment of epilepsy was discussed in earnest.

Fedor Krause was one of several neurosurgeons who spoke at the inaugural International League Against Epilepsy meeting. Soon afterward, he published an article about epilepsy surgery, signifying increased awareness of neurosurgical intervention for epilepsy.[8] Krause continued to operate on patients with epilepsy. He refined the approach pioneered by Horsley but also attempted to expand the indication for epilepsy surgery. Specifically, Krause wanted to operate not only on patients with obvious posttraumatic or tumor-based causes of epilepsy, but also on those with no discrete lesion or macroscopic pathology. His reasoning, along with his partner Schum,[9] was that if clear seizure semiology pointed to a likely location of an epileptogenic focus, then that region should be resectable. Because the most clearly characterized semiology at the time was the afore-mentioned Jacksonian march, these were the patients on whom Krause operated.[5] For those patients with Jacksonian seizures but no obvious lesion in the motor cortex, Krause used monopolar faradic stimulation along the motor cortex to induce the seizure and localize the epileptogenic focus. In doing so, he eventually mapped the motor cortex along the precentral gyrus, supporting Horsley's (and others') findings in monkeys.[7] This work provided a significant advancement in neurosurgical localization and understanding of brain function. Additionally, although not all his patients improved, Krause's work represented a significant improvement in surgical technique and held promise for advancing epilepsy surgery. Krause and Schum's[9] lengthy volume on epilepsy published in 1932 formally advocated for localization and surgical resection of epileptogenic foci even in the absence of discrete lesions.

Better understanding of brain function lent more confidence in the endeavor of understanding nonlesional epilepsy. Mirroring Krause's characterization of the motor cortex, during Harvey Cushing's brief foray into epilepsy surgery, he established the postcentral gyrus as a sensory center based on cortical stimulation of patients with focal sensorimotor seizures.[5] With this burgeoning understanding of brain function, epilepsy surgery was poised to integrate the next big development: EEG.

The Instrumental Invention of Electroencephalography: Honing in on the Mesial Temporal Lobe

The potential role of EEG in epilepsy diagnostics began to take form with the collaboration of Herbert Jasper and Wilder Penfield in the 1930s. On hearing of Jasper's advances in EEG recording at Brown University in Rhode Island (which were also informed by contemporaneous advances by Frederic Gibbs and William Lennox at Harvard),[10] Penfield was sufficiently intrigued to discuss the possibility of integrating EEG with neurosurgical treatment. Having founded the Montreal Neurological Institute (MNI) in 1934 with a keen interest in epilepsy and extensively operating on non-neoplastic epilepsy based on the ideas advanced by Krause and Schum, Penfield was cautiously optimistic about the role EEG could play in advancing the field.

The collaboration between Penfield and Jasper at the MNI proved fruitful. The work of Jasper and his colleagues established and fine-tuned the diagnostic and localizing capabilities of EEG in 1941.[11] Gibbs and Lennox, also working on EEG, went so far as to claim that nonlesional epilepsy was more common than lesional epilepsy, a bold claim at the time.[5] Further diagnostic capability was provided by intraoperative cortical surface recordings (electrocorticography [ECoG]). By 1941, it became evident that characteristic patterns of abnormal electrical activity over mesial temporal structures along with characteristic symptomatology led to the "psychomotor" seizures; today the pathology has been termed mesial temporal lobe epilepsy, which leads to complex partial seizures.[5] With electrophysiologic justification for temporal lobe pathology despite the absence of discrete lesions, surgical resection of this region seemed reasonable. Elucidation of mesial temporal function lagged, however, behind the identification of pathology. What sort of neurologic issues would be encountered if this region were to be resected? Through the 1940s, this question was addressed through the study of hippocampal and amygdala function[12] and more confidence in attempting surgical exploration resulted. Electrophysiologic studies proved useful for localization in tumoral and other lesion-based epilepsy as well.

In 1949 and 1950, with the use of EEG and ECoG, Jasper, Penfield, and Flanigan reported on multiple series of patients who had been operated on in light of diagnostic EEG findings.[5] In the first report by Jasper in 1949, 24 patients were operated on, but only 2 had had surgical resection of the uncus because of continued uncertainty about the lack of discrete structural alterations.[13] In the 1950 report by Penfield and Flanigan, however, 68 patients were operated on, of whom 10 had resection of their uncus and 2 had hippocampectomies as well.[5,14] Approximately half of these patients achieved seizure control, which provided the initial proof of principle but indicated the need for further study.

Further studies at this time led to refinements in the procedure. Histopathologic study of resected tissue by Gibbs and Percival Bailey led to better characterization of the anatomic range of microscopic pathology.[5] Electrophysiologic studies also redefined surgical goals. In particular, early case series attempted to minimize resected surface area by taking regions with maximal abnormal ECoG activity. Because seizures persisted in these patients, however, increased region of resection was practiced until the entirety of the anterior temporal lobe began to be resected.[10]

Refining Understanding and Surgical Approach

After the success of anteromesial resection, operative experience aimed at better understanding seizure propagation and the structures in the region. Intraoperative stimulation allowed these distinctions to be made. When ictal responses were induced, seizure propagation could be studied. When acute changes in memory and mood occurred, normal function of mesial temporal structures was better understood.

Armed with this understanding, Penfield and Baldwin[15] defined a standardized approach to anteromesial temporal lobe resection in 1952. This seminal approach extended more mesially than what was reported in previous case series. Through the rest of the 1950s and early 1960s, this approach was used at many other centers and reported on in more case series.[16,17] En bloc resection was also introduced by Falconer in 1953.[18] Late in the 1960s, Niemeyer and Bello of Brazil developed a selective amygdalohippocampectomy (SelAH) using a transventricular approach, which allowed preservation of some anterior temporal neocortical tissue.[19] The introduction of a selective approach was crucial for the ablative procedures of today.

With rapid innovation in surgical technique, along with improved seizure freedom outcomes in patients, surgery for epilepsy experienced a sharp rise in popularity. The 1950s saw a worldwide growth of centers practicing anterior temporal lobectomies and other procedures for epilepsy. Centers in Japan[20] and Brazil[21] (including that of Niemeyer) are a few international regions that practiced these surgeries with increasing frequency.

The Advent of Stereotaxis

While the neuroanatomic correlates of temporal lobe epilepsy, its treatment by open surgical resection, and potential selective approaches were being elucidated, the stereotactic approach to neurosurgery was also being developed. First used in 1906 in animal studies by Horsley and Clarke, the stereotactic frame is a rigid, head-mounted frame that allows for adjustments in the Cartesian X, Y, and Z planes.[22] This method of coordinate-based targeting allows specific regions of the brain to be accessed in a precise manner. With continued improvement on Horsley and Clarke's initial plaster-based fixation system, stereotactic surgery was first applied to humans in 1947. Spiegel and colleagues[23] used a stereotactic frame to perform a medial thalamotomy for a psychiatric indication. After this initial use, they actually used stereotactic surgery for some cases of

epilepsy. It was not until the 1960s, however, that further advances, including stereotactic apparatus improvement by Leksell[24] and methodological improvements by the group of Talairach and Bancaud[25] in France, allowed stereotaxis to be used in earnest for epilepsy surgery. The stereotactic approach remains central to today's ablative epilepsy surgery. After the theme of localization of structures demonstrated by targeting posttraumatic scars, tumors, and mesial temporal sclerosis, stereotaxy did much to improve the precision of epilepsy surgery in 2 important domains: diagnostics and surgical approach.

Although the domains of diagnostics and surgical approach are now interdependent, they developed separately. Stereotactic surgery for epilepsy arose initially from surgical treatment of behavioral/psychiatric disturbances. In a series by Umbach and Riechert[26] in Germany, stereotactic amygdalotomy was used in conjunction with fornicotomy, and amelioration of epileptic symptoms was an unexpected outcome. Early stereotactic epilepsy surgeries followed similar rationale, but the strict use of stereotactic surgery for epilepsy did not gain popularity until improved methods were developed. An early case series of interest was reported by Vladyka[27] in the late 1960s, who used ventriculography and a stereotactic atlas to perform stereotactic ablative amygdalotomy (by way of a thermocoagulative lesion). Results in this series were comparable to open surgery, yet, as discussed previously, stereotactic surgery for epilepsy remained largely unpopular until much later.

The use of stereotaxis for diagnostics, however, became much more prominent in the form of stereotactic EEG (SEEG). Because the only available diagnostic modalities before SEEG were noninvasive scalp EEG and ECoG, preoperative mapping of subcortical epileptogenic foci remained limited. The work of Talairach and Bancaud was instrumental in developing and refining SEEG. Choosing a different approach from Jasper and Penfield, who relied on ECoG and cortical stimulation to define the seizure, Talairach and Bancaud used seizure semiology to formulate a reasonable hypothesis about the spatial procession of the seizure through regions of the brain. They then used a crude form of stereotaxis to place multiple flexible depth electrodes in those same regions.[28] Recordings of electrical activity provided information about potential locations of epileptogenic foci in these patients. As discussed previously, however, the stereotactic approach was not commonly used for the surgical approach to the same patients. There are multiple reasons for this phenomenon. Even with the addition of SEEG, only an approximate location was provided and, moreover, there was a lack of definitive atlases for stereotactic navigation at this time. As a result, patients undergoing SEEG for MTLE through the 1960s and 1970s typically underwent open resection following standard approaches for anteromesial temporal lobectomies.[7] In the 1980s, further refinement of technique occurred, including an easier approach for placing depth electrodes in the mesial temporal lobe through the foramen ovale.[29] With better information from preoperative diagnostics, early forays into selective, microsurgical treatment of epilepsy were seen, including a 1982 report on SelAH.[30]

SEEG continued to be refined and incorporated into surgical planning. Its technical difficulty has limited its widespread expansion out of Europe, but updated techniques have been described recently.[31] The use of stereotactic surgery for epilepsy was similarly limited in spread, even with the publication of stereotactic atlases, and open resection continued to be favored through the 1980s and 1990s. Advances in neuroimaging in the 1990s, however, have allowed several stereotactic ablative procedures to join open resection as valuable tools for epilepsy surgery. The goal of ablative epilepsy surgery, for both lesional and nonlesional causes, is to offer minimal interruption of normal circuits (and, consequently, normal behavior) while offering maximal seizure control.

Other Forms of Epilepsy and Surgical Techniques

Until this point, primarily the history of the surgical approach for MTLE has been discussed because it is both the most commonly operated-on form of epilepsy and the form that inspired advances in ablative neurosurgery. Other forms of epilepsy, however, are also subject to surgical intervention. These approaches have developed over time as well. Surgical treatment of tumoral epilepsy has followed similar trends to MTLE, including craniotomy, better localization with EEG and imaging, and application of current minimally invasive techniques.[7,10] Hypothalamic hamartoma, a less common cause of intractable secondary generalized seizures, has proved more difficult to treat given its difficult location. Reports in the late 1960s used various approaches for resection,[32] but precise access has awaited development of neuroimaging and stereotactic techniques (described later). For epileptic disorders with less focal pathologic correlates, 2 important nonablative techniques are used: hemispherectomy and corpus callosotomy. The historical context of these procedures is discussed briefly.

Hemispherectomy

Initially used for treatment of malignant gliomas[33,34] in the late 1920s, hemispherectomy fell out of favor until 1938 (both for tumors and epilepsy), when it was described for epilepsy.[35] Some case series were reported in the 1950s for infantile and pediatric forms of epilepsy.[36,37] After refinements in procedure, hemispherectomy has become more of a disconnection procedure than a resective one.[38] Today, hemispherectomy is useful for multifocal, intractable seizures localized to one hemisphere. Some indications include Sturge-Weber syndrome, cortical dysplasia, and Rasmussen encephalitis.[35]

Corpus callosotomy

The corpus callosotomy was first described in a case series by William van Wagenen in 1940.[39] It was performed in 10 patients with epilepsy related to callosal gliomas, with all patients demonstrating some degree of improvement.[40] Two decades later, corpus callosotomy was used again in patients with intractable epilepsy.[39] Patient improvement led the technique to gain favor through the 1970s, and studies of hemispheric functional localization spearheaded by Sperry led to his receipt of the Nobel Prize in 1981.[39] Corpus callosotomy continues to be practiced today for intractable epilepsy from hypothalamic hamartoma and childhood epilepsies, such as Lennox-Gastaut syndrome,[41] among others.

Having completed a general overview of the history of epilepsy surgery, current technical approaches in practice and corresponding case series for these procedures are discussed.

TECHNICAL APPROACHES/CURRENT PRACTICE IN ABLATIVE EPILEPSY SURGERY
Open Approaches

Since its initial characterization, as described previously, MTL has been greatly elucidated. Given its restricted epileptogenic zone and frequent pharmacoresistance, MTLE is particularly amenable to surgical resection. As such, it is the form of epilepsy that is most commonly reported on in a surgical capacity. It is instructive to discuss open approaches, because they inform less-invasive ablative approaches. The most commonly used approaches include[42]

- Standard anteromesial temporal lobectomy (ATL), which involves resection of the anterolateral aspect of the temporal lobe demarcated at 3.5 cm from the anteriormost portion of the temporal lobe. Mesial amygdalohippocampectomy (AH) follows. This procedure is the direct descendant of the ATL that was standardized in the 1950s, as described previously. ATL can also be individualized for a specific patient based on intraoperative mapping before performing AH.

- SelAH, in which transylvian or transcortical approaches are used to access the mesial temporal lobe. On reaching these structures, AH is performed. This procedure follows from the selective approaches developed in the 1980s (discussed previously).

In 2001, a randomized controlled trial was performed comparing open ATL to best medical therapy. The investigators concluded that surgical resection was the gold standard for the management of not only treatment-refractory MTLE but also of MTLE before the failure of multiple antiepileptic drugs. Citing advances in neuroimaging and surgical technique, early surgical intervention was proposed based on the findings of 58% to 64% seizure freedom in the surgical group versus 8% in the medical therapy group after 1 year follow-up, with minimal side effects.[43] In regard to specific surgical technique, 1 study demonstrated a slight advantage to larger temporal resections preceding AH.[44]

It is possible, however, that the sparing of temporal tissue in SelAH may provide better cognitive outcomes. Lateralized adverse effects have been shown, with dominant-sided open ATL correlated with impairments in verbal learning and memory, and nondominant-sided open ATL with visual defects.[45,46] Moreover, despite carrying low morbidity and mortality, open ATL is still associated with a 0.24% chance of death, 2% chance of serious permanent complications, and 6% chance of transient complications.[46,48] Therefore, given the potential for fewer adverse effects, maintenance of cognitive ability, and a lesser invasive approach while still providing clinical benefit, stereotactic approaches to ablative epilepsy surgery have been on the rise more recently.

Stereotactic Ablative Approaches

Building on the use of stereotaxy for other intracranial procedures, such as tumors and deep brain stimulation, epilepsy surgery has seen the rapid incorporation of newer, minimally invasive methods in the past decade. These procedures have incorporated refinement of surgical technique, better instrumentation, and preoperative/intraoperative neuroimaging to markedly improve precision. Many of these procedures are discussed in greater detail by Gross and Colleagues,[47] but a brief overview of the major

stereotactic ablative epilepsy surgeries used today is provided. Before doing so, however, the evolution of ablative procedures is briefly discussed to contextualize this overview.

Evolution of ablative procedures

In 1824, Marie Jean-Pierre Flourens performed the first experimental brain ablation in mammalian species, using the technique to define brain function.[49] With development of radiofrequency ablation (RFA), in which high-frequency current is passed to induce cell death of a specific region, the first known therapeutic neurosurgical application of ablation was performed in 1931 for trigeminal neuralgia.[50] It was then applied to Parkinson disease in 1939 by Meyers.[51] Before this time, the therapeutic potential of lesioning the brain was recognized, but contemporary methods, including local alcohol injection, radioactive seeds, direct electrical current, and primitive focused ultrasound, had their drawbacks.[52] Refinements in understanding of radiofrequency lesions in the brain continued with methodological studies,[53] histologic studies,[54] and experiments to control lesion size.[55] Commercial RFA apparatus became available in the late 1950s. With better mechanistic understanding of and better equipment for the procedure, RFA began to regularly be applied to epilepsy[27] and psychiatric neurosurgery.[56] Current practice in ablative neurosurgery for epilepsy leverages advances in stereotactic techniques and alternative ablative technologies, such as radiosurgery, laser, and focused ultrasound.

Current approaches

Ablative procedures are used for both MTLE and lesional epilepsy (tumors, arteriovenous malformations, cavernous malformations, and hypothalamic hamartomas).[46] The important procedures used today include

- Stereotactic radiofrequency thermoablation (SRT)
- Magnetic resonance (MR)–guided laser-induced interstitial therapy (MRgLITT)
- Stereotactic radiosurgery (SRS)
- MR-guided transcranial focused ultrasound (MRgFUS)

Stereotactic radiofrequency thermocoagulation In SRT, a stereotactically placed monopolar needle is used to deliver high-frequency current.[46] For MTLE, the mesial temporal lobe is typically accessed via an occipital approach.[57,58] SRT also has applications for epilepsy secondary to hypothalamic hamartoma.[59,60] Incorporation of CT[61] and, more recently, MRI,[58] have improved outcomes for SRT. The technique has been proved comparable to open ATL in seizure freedom, while providing better cognitive outcomes.[62,63] Although more studies are needed, these initial case series show promising results for SRT.

Magnetic resonance–guided laser-induced interstitial therapy Using a stereotactically placed laser diode within a fiber optic catheter to deliver thermal energy for tissue ablation, MRgLITT is procedure that has been used to treat breast cancer and liver metastases in the past.[64,65] As with other stereotactic neurosurgical procedures however, recent improvements in methodology and technology have cultivated the neurosurgical application of MRgLITT. An important development in MRgLITT has been the incorporation of MR thermometry, which provides real-time feedback of the temperature of the region being ablated. This added level of monitoring provides further precision of treatment. Also used for the treatment of recurrent brain tumors,[66–68] MRgLITT has been used for MTLE with good results.[69,70] MRgLITT continues to be studied. With characterization of imaging changes in epilepsy[71] and details of the technique itself,[72] along with further case series, the technique promises to be a valuable option for treating MTLE.

Stereotactic radiosurgery The stereotactic, noninvasive delivery of ionizing radiation to a specific target defines SRS. This form of ablation can be mediated by Gamma Knife (most commonly), CyberKnife, or linear accelerators.[46] SRS has a long history of applications to lesional epilepsy, including tumors,[73] arteriovenous malformations,[74] and hypothalamic hamartomas.[75] It has also been used for psychiatric indications since the 1970s.

SRS was first reported for MTLE in 1995. Multiple studies since then have shown a heterogeneous treatment effect due to variables, such as dose and patient selection.[46] In regard to the former, different studies have used low-dose protocols whereas others have used high-dose protocols. The latter seems more efficacious,[76] although the exact protocol needs further delineation. Moreover, given the highly selective nature of the AH mediated by SRS, patients must absolutely demonstrate proper mesial temporal epileptic pathophysiology.[46] This strict patient selection, which holds for all other surgical approaches, ensures that maximal therapeutic effect can be achieved. SRS, similar to the other minimally invasive stereotactic approaches discussed, also provides better cognitive outcomes than open ATL.[77] As such, it continues to be used and refined.

Magnetic resonance–guided transcranial focused ultrasound Although not used for MTLE yet, MRgFUS is a promising therapy with current applications in the treatment of glioblastoma,[78] chronic pain,[79,80] and essential tremor.[80,81] The focal ablative lesions of MRgFUS are mediated by focused, high-frequency sound waves.[82] As with MRgLITT, MR guidance aids the precision of focusing. Current advances in MRgFUS have actually made it an entirely noninvasive procedure (the former incarnation required a craniotomy). Currently, however, the technology is limited in its ability to access mesial temporal structures.[46] These issues are being studied, and MRgFUS holds promise for the future treatment of MTLE.

SUMMARY

The idea of neurosurgery for epilepsy began in antiquity with the use of trephination. The birth of analytical clinical neurology with Hughlings Jackson motivated meticulous characterization of seizure semiology, leading to justification for craniotomies. Refinement in technique followed, but the major development of EEG allowed Jasper, Penfield, Gibbs, Lennox, and other investigators to understand electrical manifestations of pathologic activity in the brain. In this manner, epilepsy surgery broadened its scope from posttraumatic scars and tumors to include nonlesional epilepsy. MTLE was characterized and its surgical treatment standardized in the 1950s in the form of the ATLs. With the advent of stereotaxis in the 1960s, better understanding of the pathophysiology of MTLE followed, and more informed surgical choices were made. The first inklings of selective approaches of resecting only amygdala and hippocampus appeared in the late 1970s. Further refinement of these approaches, along with the extension of stereotaxis from the domain of preoperative diagnostics to that of bona fide epilepsy surgery, followed the development of neuroimaging. Currently, open ATL is still considered the gold standard. Newer, minimally invasive methods, however, have been better characterized, including SRT, MRgLITT, SRT, and MRgFUS. These methods seem to promise seizure freedom rates similar to open ATL with less cognitive impairment.

The eminent physician William Osler, often regarded as the father of modern medicine, was characteristically prescient in his observations about the emerging field of neurosurgery in 1907:

> …[I] would prefer to see neurology a special department so that there would not be neurological physicians and surgeons, but

medico-chirurgical neurologists, properly trained in the anatomical, physiological, clinical and surgical aspects of the subject.[5,83]

Osler would have appreciated the development of epilepsy surgery. Its history is rife with instances of neurosurgeons practicing neurology, neurologists incorporating neurosurgical techniques into their repertoire, and the potent collaboration between and integration of the fields. Today, stereotactic, minimally invasive surgical techniques and more precise electrophysiologic understanding integrate neurosurgery, neurology, engineering, and electrophysiology to precisely localize epileptogenic foci. These approaches seem to minimize adverse cognitive effects while maintaining therapeutic efficacy seen in open approaches. From modest beginnings in antiquity with trephination, to the first craniotomies for epilepsy by Horsley, to the collaboration of Jasper and Penfield, and to all the contributors along the way, epilepsy surgery has advanced significantly in the past 150 years. With current advances, it promises to continue offering better relief to those suffering from a devastating, debilitating disorder.

REFERENCES

1. Wolf P. History of epilepsy: nosological concepts and classification. Epileptic Disord 2014;16:261–9.
2. Uff C, Frith D, Harrison C, et al. Sir Victor Horsley's 19th century operations at the national hospital for neurology and neurosurgery, queen square. J Neurosurg 2010;114:534–42.
3. York GK, Steinberg DA. Hughlings Jackson's neurological ideas. Brain 2011;134:3106–13.
4. Jackson JH. A study of convulsions. Trans St Andrews Med Grad Assoc 1869;45:412–6.
5. Feindel W, Leblanc R, De Almeida AN. Epilepsy surgery: historical highlights 1909–2009. Epilepsia 2009;50:131–51.
6. Horsley V. Brain surgery. BMJ 1886;2:670–5.
7. Wolf P. The history of surgical treatment of epilepsy in Europe. In: Hans Otto Lüders, editor. Epilepsy surgery. 1st edition. New York: Raven Press; 1992. p. 9–19.
8. Krause F. Die operative behandlung der epilepsie. Med Klin Berl 1909;5:1418–22.
9. Krause F, Schum H. Die spezielle Chirurgie der Gehirnkrankheiten, 2. Stuttgart (Germany): Enke; 1931.
10. Flanigin H, Hermann B, King D, et al. The history of surgical treatment of epilepsy in North America prior to 1975. In: Hans Otto Lüders, editor. Epilepsy surgery. New York: Raven Press; 1992. p. 19–37.
11. Jasper H, Kershman J. Electroencephalographic classification of the epilepsies. Arch Neurol Psychiatr 1941;45:903–43.
12. Penfield W, Milner B. Memory deficit produced by bilateral lesions in the hippocampal zone. AMA Arch Neurol Psychiatry 1958;79:475–97.
13. Jasper H. Étude anatomo-physiologique des epilepsies. In: Fischgold H, editor. Compte-rendus de 2ème Congrès International d'EEG. Paris: Masson; 1949. p. 99–111.
14. Penfield W, Flanigin H. Surgical therapy of temporal lobe seizures. AMA Arch Neurol Psychiatry 1950;64: 491–500.
15. Penfield W, Baldwin M. Temporal lobe seizures and the technic of subtotal temporal lobectomy. Ann Surg 1952;136:625–34.
16. MORRIS AA. Temporal lobectomy with removal of uncus, hippocampus, and amygdala: results for psychomotor epilepsy three to nine years after operation. AMA Arch Neurol Psychiatry 1956;76: 479–96.
17. Baldwin M, Bailey P. Temporal lobe epilepsy. Springfield (MA): Charles C. Thomas; 1958.
18. Falconer M. Discussion on the surgery of temporal lobe epilepsy: surgical and pathological results. Proc R Soc Med 1953;76:971–4.
19. Niemeyer P, Bello H. Amygdalohippocampectomy in temporal lobe epilepsy. Microsurgical technique. Excerpta Medica 1973;293:20(abstr 48).
20. Seino M, Mihara T. The history of surgical treatment of epilepsy in Japan. In: Hans Otto Lüders, editor. Epilepsy surgery. 1st edition. New York: Raven Press; 1992. p. 37–40.
21. Godoy J. The history of surgical treatment of epilepsy in South America. In: Hans Otto Lüders, editor. Epilepsy surgery. 1st edition. New York: Raven Press; 1992. p. 41–4.
22. Pereira EAC, Green AL, Nandi D, et al. Stereotactic neurosurgery in the United Kingdom: the hundred years from Horsley to Hariz. Neurosurgery 2008; 63:594–606 [discussion: 606–7].
23. Spiegel EA, Wycis HT, Marks M, et al. Stereotaxic apparatus for operations on the human brain. Science 1947;106:349–50.
24. Leksell L. A stereotactic apparatus for intracerebral surgery. Acta Chir Scand 1949;99:229–33.
25. Talairach J, Bancaud J, Szikla G, et al. Approche nouvelle de la neurochirurgie de l'epilepsie. Méthodologie stéréotaxique et résultats thérapeutiques. Neurochirurgie 1974;20(Suppl 1):1–274.
26. Umbach W, Riechert T. Elektrophysiologische und klinische Ergebnisse stereotaktischer Eingriffe im limbischen System bei temporaler Epilepsie. Nervenarzt 1964;35:482–8.
27. Vladyka V. Tactics in surgical treatment of epilepsy and its realization in cases of temporal epilepsy. Cesk Slov Neurol Neurochir 1978;41:95–106.
28. Kahane P, Landré E, Minotti L, et al. The Bancaud and Talairach view on the epileptogenic zone: a working hypothesis. Epileptic Disord 2006;

8(Suppl 2):S16–26. Erratum in: Epileptic Disord 2008;10(2):191. PubMed PMID: 17012069.

29. Wieser HG, Elger CE, Stodieck SR. The 'foramen ovale electrode': a new recording method for the preoperative evaluation of patients suffering from mesio-basal temporal lobe epilepsy. Electroencephalogr Clin Neurophysiol 1985;61:314–22.

30. Wieser HG, Yaşargil MG. Selective amygdalohippocampectomy as a surgical treatment of mesiobasal limbic epilepsy. Surg Neurol 1982;17:445–57.

31. Gonzalez-Martinez J, Mullin J, Vadera S, et al. Stereotactic placement of depth electrodes in medically intractable epilepsy. J Neurosurg 2014;120: 639–44.

32. Rosenfeld JV. The evolution of treatment for hypothalamic hamartoma: a personal odyssey. Neurosurg Focus 2011;30:E1.

33. Dandy WE. Removal of right cerebral hemisphere for certain tumors with hemiplegia: preliminary report. J Am Med Assoc 1928;90:823–5.

34. Gardner W. Removal of the right cerebral hemisphere for infiltrating glioma: report of a case. J Am Med Assoc 1933;101:823–6.

35. Beier AD, Rutka JT. Hemispherectomy: historical review and recent technical advances. Neurosurg Focus 2013;34:E11.

36. Hendrick EB, Hoffman HJ, Hudson AR. Hemispherectomy in children. Clin Neurosurg 1969;16:315–27.

37. Krynauw RA. Infantile hemiplegia treated by removing one cerebral hemisphere. J Neurol Neurosurg Psychiatry 1950;13:243–67.

38. De Ribaupierre S, Delalande O. Hemispherotomy and other disconnective techniques. Neurosurg Focus 2008;25:E14.

39. Mathews MS, Linskey ME, Binder DK. William P. van Wagenen and the first corpus callosotomies for epilepsy. J Neurosurg 2008;108:608–13.

40. van Wagenen WP, Herren R. Surgical division of commissural pathways in the corpus callosum: relation to spread of an epileptic attack. Arch Neurol Psychiatry 1940;44:740–59.

41. VanStraten AF, Ng Y-T. Update on the management of Lennox-Gastaut syndrome. Pediatr Neurol 2012; 47:153–61.

42. Gross RE, Mahmoudi B, Riley JP. Less is more: novel less-invasive surgical techniques for mesial temporal lobe epilepsy that minimize cognitive impairment. Curr Opin Neurol 2015;28:182–91.

43. Wiebe S, Blume WT, Girvin JP, et al, Effectiveness and Efficiency of Surgery for Temporal Lobe Epilepsy Study Group. A randomized, controlled trial of surgery for temporal-lobe epilepsy. N Engl J Med 2001;345:311–8.

44. Hu W-H, Zhang C, Zhang K, et al. Selective amygdalohippocampectomy versus anterior temporal lobectomy in the management of mesial temporal lobe epilepsy: a meta-analysis of comparative studies. J Neurosurg 2013;119: 1089–97.

45. Stroup E, Langfitt J, Berg M, et al. Predicting verbal memory decline following anterior temporal lobectomy (ATL). Neurology 2003;60:1266–73.

46. Quigg M, Harden C. Minimally invasive techniques for epilepsy surgery: stereotactic radiosurgery and other technologies. J Neurosurg 2014;121(Suppl): 232–40.

47. Gross RE, Willie JT, Drane DL. The Role of Stereotactic Laser Amygdalohippocampotomy in Mesial Temporal Lobe Epilepsy. Neurosurg Clin N Am 2015, in press.

48. Thom M, Mathern GW, Cross JH, et al. Mesial temporal lobe epilepsy: how do we improve surgical outcome? Ann Neurol 2010;68:424–34.

49. Yildirim FB, Sarikcioglu L. Marie Jean Pierre Flourens (1794–1867): an extraordinary scientist of his time. J Neurol Neurosurg Psychiatry 2007;78:852.

50. Soloman M, Mekhail MN, Mekhail N. Radiofrequency treatment in chronic pain. Expert Rev Neurother 2010;10:469–74.

51. Turner DA. Modern neurosurgery: clinical translation of neuroscience advances. Florence (KY): CRC Press; 2004.

52. Aronow S. The use of radio-frequency power in making lesions in the brain. J Neurosurg 1960;17: 431–8.

53. Organ LW. Electrophysiologic principles of radiofrequency lesion making. Appl Neurophysiol 1976;39: 69–76.

54. Åström K-E. The pathology of artificially produced lesions in the central nervous system. Acta Neurol Scand 1963;39:127–38.

55. Watkins ES. Heat Gains in Brain During Electrocoagulative Lesions. J Neurosurg 1965;23:319–28.

56. Sinha S, McGovern RA, Mikell CB, et al. Ablative limbic system surgery: review and future directions. Curr Behav Neurosci Rep 2015;2(2):49–59.

57. Liscak R, Malikova H, Kalina M, et al. Stereotactic radiofrequency amygdalohippocampectomy in the treatment of mesial temporal lobe epilepsy. Acta Neurochir (Wien) 2010;152:1291–8.

58. Vojtěch Z, Malíková H, Krámská L, et al. MRI-guided stereotactic amygdalohippocampectomy: a single center experience. Neuropsychiatr Dis Treat 2015; 11:359–74.

59. Fujimoto Y, Kato A, Saitoh Y, et al. Open radiofrequency ablation for the management of intractable epilepsy associated with sessile hypothalamic hamartoma. Minim Invasive Neurosurg 2005;48: 132–5.

60. Wang W, Wang W, Guo X, et al. Hypothalamic hamartoma causing gelastic seizures treated with stereotactic radiofrequency thermocoagulation. Epileptic Disord Int Epilepsy J Videotape 2009;11: 333–8.

61. Patil AA, Andrews R, Torkelson R. Stereotactic volumetric radiofrequency lesioning of intracranial structures for control of intractable seizures. Stereotact Funct Neurosurg 1995;64:123–33.

62. Malikova H, Kramska L, Vojtech Z, et al. Stereotactic radiofrequency amygdalohippocampectomy: two years of good neuropsychological outcomes. Epilepsy Res 2013;106:423–32.

63. Malikova H, Kramska L, Vojtech Z, et al. Different surgical approaches for mesial temporal epilepsy: resection extent, seizure, and neuropsychological outcomes. Stereotact Funct Neurosurg 2014;92: 372–80.

64. Van Esser S, Stapper G, van Diest PJ, et al. Ultrasound-guided laser-induced thermal therapy for small palpable invasive breast carcinomas: a feasibility study. Ann Surg Oncol 2009;16:2259–63.

65. Vogl TJ, Mack M, Eichler K, et al. Effect of laser-induced thermotherapy on liver metastases. Expert Rev Anticancer Ther 2006;6:769–74.

66. Jethwa PR, Barrese JC, Gowda A, et al. Magnetic resonance thermometry-guided laser-induced thermal therapy for intracranial neoplasms: initial experience. Neurosurgery 2012;71:133–44, 144–5.

67. Kahn T, Bettag M, Ulrich F, et al. MRI-guided laser-induced interstitial thermotherapy of cerebral neoplasms. J Comput Assist Tomogr 1994;18:519–32.

68. Torres-Reveron J, Tomasiewicz HC, Shetty A, et al. Stereotactic laser induced thermotherapy (LITT): a novel treatment for brain lesions regrowing after radiosurgery. J Neurooncol 2013;113:495–503.

69. Curry DJ, Gowda A, McNichols RJ, et al. MR-guided stereotactic laser ablation of epileptogenic foci in children. Epilepsy Behav 2012;24:408–14.

70. Willie JT, Laxpati NG, Drane DL, et al. Real-time magnetic resonance-guided stereotactic laser amygdalohippocampotomy for mesial temporal lobe epilepsy. Neurosurgery 2014;74:569–85.

71. Tiwari P, Danish S, Wong S, et al. Quantitative evaluation of multi-parametric MR imaging marker changes post-laser interstitial ablation therapy (LITT) for epilepsy. Proc SPIE Int Soc Opt Eng 2013;8671:86711y.

72. Sinha S, Hargreaves E, Patel NV, et al. Assessment of irrigation dynamics in magnetic-resonance guided laser induced thermal therapy (MRgLITT). Lasers Surg Med 2015;47:273–80.

73. Schröttner O, Eder HG, Unger F, et al. Radiosurgery in lesional epilepsy: brain tumors. Stereotact Funct Neurosurg 1998;70(Suppl 1):50–6.

74. Steiner L, Lindquist C, Adler JR, et al. Clinical outcome of radiosurgery for cerebral arteriovenous malformations. J Neurosurg 1992;77:1–8.

75. Régis J, Scavarda D, Tamura M, et al. Epilepsy related to hypothalamic hamartomas: surgical management with special reference to gamma knife surgery. Childs Nerv Syst 2006;22:881–95.

76. Chang EF, Quigg M, Oh MC, et al. Predictors of efficacy after stereotactic radiosurgery for medial temporal lobe epilepsy. Neurology 2010;74:165–72.

77. Régis J, Rey M, Bartolomei F, et al. Gamma knife surgery in mesial temporal lobe epilepsy: a prospective multicenter study. Epilepsia 2004;45: 504–15.

78. McDannold N, Clement GT, Black P, et al. Transcranial magnetic resonance imaging- guided focused ultrasound surgery of brain tumors: initial findings in 3 patients. Neurosurgery 2010;66:323–32 [discussion: 332].

79. Martin E, Jeanmonod D, Morel A, et al. High-intensity focused ultrasound for noninvasive functional neurosurgery. Ann Neurol 2009;66:858–61.

80. Jung HH, Chang WS, Rachmilevitch I, et al. Different magnetic resonance imaging patterns after transcranial magnetic resonance-guided focused ultrasound of the ventral intermediate nucleus of the thalamus and anterior limb of the internal capsule in patients with essential tremor or obsessive-compulsive disorder. J Neurosurg 2015; 122:162–8.

81. Elias WJ, Huss D, Voss T, et al. A pilot study of focused ultrasound thalamotomy for essential tremor. N Engl J Med 2013;369:640–8.

82. Jolesz FA, Hynynen K, McDannold N, et al. MR imaging-controlled focused ultrasound ablation: a noninvasive image-guided surgery. Magn Reson Imaging Clin N Am 2005;13:545–60.

83. Feindel W. Osler and the 'medico-chirurgical neurologists': horsley, cushing, and penfield. J Neurosurg 2003;99:188–99.

The Role of Stereotactic Laser Amygdalohippocampotomy in Mesial Temporal Lobe Epilepsy

Robert E. Gross, MD, PhD[a,b,c,d,]*, Jon T. Willie, MD, PhD[a,b,c],
Daniel L. Drane, PhD[b,e]

KEYWORDS

- Mesial temporal lobe epilepsy • Mesial temporal sclerosis • Laser • Anterior temporal lobectomy
- Selective amygdalohippocampectomy • Ablation • Neuropsychology • Memory

KEY POINTS

- Stereotactic laser amygdalohippocampotomy (SLAH) is a minimally invasive approach to the treatment of medication-resistant mesial temporal lobe epilepsy that accomplishes ablation of the seizure focus with real-time magnetic resonance thermal mapping.
- Seizure-free rates in early series suggest that SLAH approaches the effectiveness of open resection for patients with mesial temporal sclerosis (MTS).
- SLAH avoids neurocognitive adverse effects of open resection on naming (dominant side) and object recognition (nondominant side).
- Although early data suggest more preserved memory function after SLAH, further research is required. Thus, patients with relatively preserved memory in the absence of MTS are offered SLAH only after careful considerations of risks, benefits, and alternative procedures, including neuromodulation.
- Secondary benefits of SLAH include decreased length of stay, elimination of intensive care unit stay, reduced procedure-related discomfort, and improved access to surgical treatment for patients less likely to consider an open resective procedure.

 Video of laser ablation accompanies this article at www.neurosurgery.theclinics.com/

Disclosures: Funding was provided to Emory University by way of a clinical study agreement from Visualase, which developed products related to the research described in this article. In addition, R.E. Gross served as a consultant to Visualase and Medtronic and received compensation for these services. The terms of this arrangement have been reviewed and approved by Emory University in accordance with its conflict of interest policies. D.L. Drane receives funding from the NIH/NINDS (K02 NS070960), which provides support for his work.
[a] Department of Neurosurgery, Emory University School of Medicine, 1365 Clifton Road N.E., Atlanta, GA 30322, USA; [b] Department of Neurology, Emory University School of Medicine, 101 Woodruff Circle, Suite 6111, Atlanta, GA 30322, USA; [c] Interventional MRI Program, Emory University Hospital, 1364 Clifton Road, N.E., Atlanta, GA 30322, USA; [d] Coulter Department of Biomedical Engineering, Emory University, 1760 Haygood Dr, Ste W 200, Atlanta, GA 30322, USA; [e] Department of Neurology, University of Washington School of Medicine, Harborview Medical Center, 325 9th Avenue, Seattle, WA 98104, USA
* Corresponding author. Department of Neurosurgery, Emory University School of Medicine, 1365 Clifton Road, Northeast, Suite 6200, Atlanta, GA 30322.
E-mail address: rgross@emory.edu

INTRODUCTION

Mesial temporal lobe epilepsy (MTLE) is the most common cause of medication-resistant epilepsy, and decades of targeted drug discovery in epilepsy have not decreased the percentage of patients with MTLE suffering disabling seizures. For these patients, resective surgical treatment, as shown in a recent meta-analysis, leads to approximately 75% of patients becoming seizure free.[1] The adverse surgical effects of open resection, whether anterior temporal lobectomy (ATL) or selective amygdalohippocampectomy (SAH), may be well tolerated in most circumstances. In the absence of other options, it has been emphasized that the benefits of seizure freedom outweigh the adverse effects, resulting in overall improvement in quality of life.[2] Nevertheless, both ATL and SAH have significant effects on neurocognitive function(s), some related to the mesial resection (eg, declarative memory impairment), but some more related to the surgical approach to the mesial structures, that is, anterior-lateral temporal resection, division, or retraction during ATL or SAH.[3–5] Cognitive declines related to the approach (collateral damage) impair naming and verbal learning (dominant hemisphere) or object recognition and figural learning (nondominant hemisphere). These impairments can be impactful and permanent, although the seizures become a distant memory. The potential of alternative, minimally invasive stereotactic procedures to accomplish the therapeutic goal of preventing seizures in the absence of such collateral damage may therefore increase the quality of life in surgical MTLE patients compared with traditional open resective procedures.

Stereotactic approaches to the mesial temporal lobe hold the promise of target ablation in the absence of collateral damage by avoiding injury as a result of the approach to the mesial temporal structures (**Table 1**). Several techniques have been explored over the last several decades.

With respect to stereotactic radiofrequency ablation (SRFA):

- Parrent and Blume[6] achieved a rate of 27% (4 of 15) seizure freedom in a subgroup of patients with many confluent lesions within the amygdala and hippocampus from a transtemporal approach, orthogonal to the hippocampal long axis, spanning 21.5 mm (mean) of the hippocampus.
- More recently, Liscak and colleagues[7] working in the Czech Republic reported seizure-free rates of 78%, comparable with open resection, by using an occipital approach along the axis of the hippocampus and a string electrode that provides more extensive lesions radial to that axis. Longer (35 mm mean) and wider ablation zones, resulting from 16 to 38 lesions (mean 25), likely contributed to the increased success rate.

Noting the recently reported successes with SRFA, we explored the use of laser interstitial thermal therapy (LITT) for MTLE. During LITT, laser light is delivered fiber-optically into tissue (interstitial) via a stereotactic approach, where photonic energy causes local heating and thermocoagulation.[8,9] Several critical advances have made modern LITT platforms into elegant and powerful neurosurgical tools (**Box 1**). The most critical advance is the ability to use MRI thermometry to

---

Table 1
Stereotactic ablation techniques

Technique	Pros	Cons
SRFA	Reduced collateral damage Immediate benefit Low cost	Temperature monitored only at tip Best results with string electrode not available in United States
Stereotactic radiosurgery (SRS)	Noninvasive	Delayed benefit after initial increase in seizures/risk of sudden unexpected death from epilepsy Potential radiation injury, dose limitations High cost
Laser interstitial thermal therapy (LITT)	Minimal collateral damage Immediate benefit Near real-time magnetic resonance thermography guides therapy and confirms ablation zone	High cost/disposables

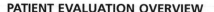

> **Box 1**
> **Laser interstitial thermal therapy**
>
> - Optical fiber with diffusing tip (10 or 3 mm)
> - Cooling cannula to control thermal spread within tissue and protect device tip
> - 984-nm diode laser causes rapid heating of water within tissue
> - Magnetic resonance thermography reads temperature change in all voxels
> - Six safety points to automatically shut off laser if temperature limits exceeded
> - Irreversible damage zone estimate at each voxel based on Arrhenius equation

measure not only the temperature at the device tip (the only temperature monitored in radiofrequency [RF] ablation) but also the temperature of tissue any distance from the tip during heating, thus providing near real-time confirmation of the ablation zone relative to off-target structures.

The mechanism of heating, that is, photonic, is different from RF ablation, but the effects of temperature on tissue are the same (**Fig. 1**). However, with LITT, magnetic resonance (MR) thermography allows temperature monitoring beyond the laser tip, whereas in RF the thermocouple provides only temperature adjacent to the device tip. This technology allows protection of off-target tissue at risk in a way that is not possible with standard use of RF ablation. At present, 2 LITT devices are available in the United States that offer overlapping but distinctive features, only one of which (Visualase, Medtronic, Louisville, CO) we have used in our studies.

PATIENT EVALUATION OVERVIEW

Patients undergoing LITT for thermocoagulation of the mesial temporal structures, which we termed stereotactic laser amygdalohippocampotomy (SLAH),[10] undergo the standard workup of patients being considered for epilepsy surgery, and our criteria are similar to those for the recommendation of open resective surgery (**Box 2**). In this article, that evaluation is reviewed as it pertains specifically to SLAH. Our decision tree is described later; extensive discussion of indications for mesial temporal lobe surgery is beyond the scope of this article.

History

A careful history of medication usage is sufficient to identify medication-resistant epilepsy, defined as "failure of adequate trials of two tolerated, appropriately chosen, and used antiepileptic drug schedules (whether as monotherapies or in combination) to achieve sustained seizure freedom."[11] A history of typical mesial temporal lobe seizure semiology (dyscognitive) with or without aura is key; semiology suggestive of other onset zone(s) (eg, nighttime motor seizures suggesting frontal onsets) warrants additional investigation.

MRI Studies

MRI is sufficient to classify the presence or absence of mesial temporal sclerosis (MTS) and also to detect/exclude confounding lesions such as focal cortical dysplasias, secondary cortical gliosis, or other lesions that may indicate dual disease, a situation not uncommon in the temporal pole region.[12]

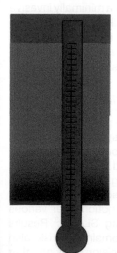

>100° C
Vaporization of intracellular and extracellular water. Rupture of cell membranes.

60° – 100° C
Instant denaturation of proteins and cellular components. Tissue coagulation.

44° – 59° C
Time-dependent thermal damage. Thermal denaturation of critical enzymes; cell death.

43° C
Critical temperature below which thermal damage does not occur regardless of exposure time.

Fig. 1. Effects of temperature on tissues. Both laser ablation and RF ablation have effects on tissues as a function of temperature. Lower than 44°C, tissue effects are absent irrespective of time. Damage is time dependent between 44°C and 59°C; damage occurs as a function of time and temperature as predicted by the Arrhenius equation. This is the important temperature range for controllable lesions using LITT. At 60°C or greater, tissue coagulation is instantaneous; these temperature effects occur close to the laser fiber diffuser tip. Instant vaporization occurs greater than 100°C; the system is generally set to turn off automatically if the temperature near the tip reaches 90°C to prevent damage to the tip.

Box 2
Criteria for candidacy for stereotactic laser amygdalohippocampotomy

- Semiology: dyscognitive seizures consistent with mesial temporal onset, ± aura (typically smell, epigastric sensation, fear, déjà vu)
- MRI: mesial temporal sclerosis positive (MTS+) or negative (MTS−)
- PET: temporal lobe hypometabolism lateralized or greater on the same side as electroencephalography
- Long-term video electroencephalographic monitoring: localization to anterior temporal region (eg, F7/T1 or F8/T2)
- Neuropsychological testing: the following refers to normally organized memory function
  - ○ MTS+ or MTS−: domain-specific memory decline present on side of anticipated ablation
  - ○ In absence of domain-specific memory decline referable to side of ablation:
    - ■ MTS+: acceptable. If memory loss is asymmetric to contralateral side, intracarotid amobarbital test (ie, Wada test) is considered
    - ■ MTS−:
      - Absence of visuospatial memory decline for nondominant ablation acceptable for ablation
      - Absence of verbal memory decline for dominant-side surgery: consider also nonablative surgical options (eg, responsive neurostimulation)
- Intracranial electroencephalography (iEEG): in setting of ambiguity as to seizure onset zone from noninvasive studies alone, onsets with iEEG referable to ipsilateral mesial temporal lobe and absence of contralateral onsets

---

Metabolic and Blood Flow Imaging

Metabolic imaging (ie, fluorodeoxyglucose-PET [FDG-PET]) is not mandatory in the setting of unilateral MTS and concordant long-term video electroencephalographic [EEG] monitoring (LTVM; see later discussion). It is corroborative when bilateral MTS is present and should be concordant with LTVM; discrepancy should prompt consideration of intracranial EEG (iEEG) monitoring. We require FDG-PET unilateral hypometabolism in non-MTS cases, which, when concordant with LTVM, may allow proceeding directly to SLAH without iEEG monitoring in nondominant cases. However, we do maintain a low threshold for iEEG in non-MTS cases. We do not routinely require subtractive ictal/interictal single-photon emission computed tomography (CT), receptor imaging, or magnetoencephalography, except in diagnostically challenging cases.

Electrographic Studies

LTVM with scalp electrodes is often sufficient to recognize the seizure onset zone in the anteromesial temporal lobe and allows for qualitative and quantitative analysis of interictal epileptiform discharges. In situations in which the seizure onset is obscured or when questions of false lateralization or bilateral onsets arise, iEEG monitoring is used. We typically use depth electrodes inserted orthogonally to provide lateral and mesial temporal coverage. Additional depth electrodes may be required to investigate other regions of interest. In certain cases, percutaneous foramen ovale electrodes may be sufficient to clarify onset laterality but should not be used alone when there is a question of lateral versus mesial or temporal versus extratemporal onsets. We insert depth electrodes through anchor bolts using standard stereotactic techniques (eg, stereotactic head frame or robotic articulating arm) to minimize the skin opening. In anticipation of the possibility of a minimally invasive therapeutic procedure, we make every attempt to similarly provide a minimally invasive diagnostic procedure (ie, minimizing the use of subdural strip and grid electrodes when possible).

Neuropsychometric Evaluation

All patients undergo extensive preoperative evaluation by specialized neuropsychologists. These tests are used both to contribute to confirmation of the onset zone as reflected in relative areas of neurocognitive weakness (eg, material specific memory dysfunction) and also to prognosticate regarding potential loss of function after various surgical approaches, including SLAH.[13] Results with respect to cognitive domains at risk also contribute to procedural decision making, that is, destructive versus nondestructive (neuromodulatory) therapeutic procedures. Further, change from baseline after surgery is informative both academically and clinically and guides referral for cognitive rehabilitation when indicated. Intracarotid amobarbital testing or the Wada test is performed on a case-by-case basis, as described later.[14]

PHARMACOLOGIC TREATMENT OPTIONS

Patients who are candidates for surgical procedures in epilepsy must be determined to be medication resistant, that is, they have tried at least 2 appropriately chosen drugs, appropriately used, and have not become seizure free.[11] After 2 failed antiepileptic drug (AED) trials, Brodie and colleagues[15–17] found that a third trial achieved only 8% and a fourth trial 4% long-term seizure freedom. However, this finding was recently re-evaluated in a larger cohort, in which 18.5% and 16.5% were made seizure free with a third and fourth AED, respectively, and decreased to 0% after 5 or 6 previous AED failures.[18] This re-evaluation of seizure intractability warrants consideration in terms of surgical options. In the setting of MTS in which the seizure-free rate is high and the risk low after both ablative and resective surgery, surgery may be considered earlier, that is, after 2 drug failures.[19] Conversely, when the chance of seizure freedom after surgery is possibly lower, such as in the absence of MTS, and risk is correspondingly higher in the setting of preserved neurocognitive functions, surgical treatment with SLAH or resection might be delayed until after a more exhaustive regimen of AEDs or neuromodulation (discussed later) have been attempted.[18]

NONPHARMACOLOGIC TREATMENT OPTIONS

For patients with MTLE, there are other, albeit less effective, treatment alternatives to open resection and laser ablation. Both vagus nerve stimulation (VNS) and responsive neurostimulation (RNS) are approved by the US Food and Drug Administration, and anterior thalamic deep brain stimulation is approved in many countries and likely pending in the United States.[20,21] These are options for patients considered poorer surgical (ie, resection or ablation) candidates, but none achieves the greater rates of seizure freedom associated with destructive surgery. We thus reserve neuromodulation for patients with MTLE in whom (1) onsets are bilateral or (2) onsets are unilateral from the dominant mesial temporal lobe and in whom verbal memory function is intact and conferred by that hemisphere. In particular, this situation occurs

typically in the setting of the hippocampus that appears normal on MRI. When verbal memory is preserved in patients with dominant-side MTS, this domain is presumed to be conferred by the contralateral hemisphere and such patients remain ablation candidates. If clarification of this situation is sought, an asymmetric Wada test result showing relative weakness of the targeted versus the nontargeted side is reassuring (see later discussion and **Fig. 2**).

SURGICAL TREATMENT OPTIONS

The decision tree regarding surgical options (see **Fig. 2**) begins with candidacy for a mesial temporal resective or ablative procedure as determined by a comprehensive epilepsy team based on the diagnostic tests outlined earlier, the most pivotal factor being the presence or absence of MTS on MRI.

Patients with Mesial Temporal Sclerosis

MRI evidence of MTS has been recognized as an important factor in selecting patients with MTLE for resective surgery,[1] and seizure freedom may be lower in patients in the absence of MTS.[22] Our results, although limited with respect to patients who do not have MTS, support similarly higher rates of seizure freedom after SLAH in patients with MTS.[10] Thus, patients with unilateral MTS and video EEG scalp monitoring providing electrographic evidence of unilateral ictal onsets confined to the anteromesial temporal lobe are excellent candidates for SLAH, with the following caveats:

1. The presence of contralateral ictal onsets or interictal spikes (a risk factor for surgical failure in open resection patients as well[22]) prompts invasive monitoring to rule out bilateral onsets or false lateralization. In the setting of well-documented bilateral ictal temporal onsets, we generally offer RNS[23] as a first-line procedure, considering unilateral SLAH for palliation if this is not feasible/desirable.
2. FDG-PET, if performed, should show concordant or predominantly ipsilateral temporal hypometabolism.
3. We use the intracarotid amobarbital (Wada) test to probe the ability of the contralateral hemisphere to support memory only in the presence of evidence that it is compromised, such as when there is more than mild visual memory loss (nondominant hemisphere function) in a dominant-side onset case, and vice versa. In the setting of a failed Wada test (inability of the contralateral hemisphere to support memory function), if there is a question of cross

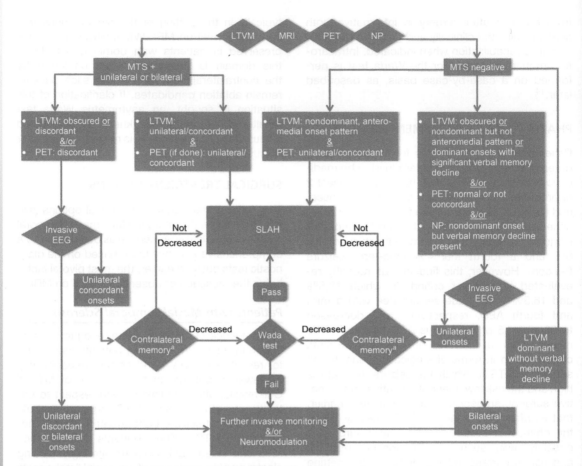

Fig. 2. Decision tree for SLAH in patients with MTLE. All patients undergo comprehensive diagnostic evaluation for epilepsy, including history, seizure semiology, MRI, fluorodeoxyglucose-PET, LTVM, and neuropsychological testing (NP). Other diagnostic tests are performed as indicated. Therapeutic decision making occurs during comprehensive epilepsy surgery conference. This decision tree is a general guide to determine surgical candidacy and may vary from case to case depending on individual patient information. [a] Depicted is the indication for Wada testing for the purpose of determining contralateral memory performance, that is, nondominant associated visual memory when the focus is on the dominant side, and vice versa. However, Wada testing is almost always performed with bilateral carotid amobarbital injections, to also determine ipsilateral memory performance that may factor into decision making as well.

flow to the contralateral internal carotid artery, we may repeat the test with an ipsilateral injection in the posterior cerebral artery (so-called selective Wada) but otherwise give strong consideration to a neuromodulation procedure (eg, VNS or RNS) rather than SLAH, irrespective of side.

4. As with resection, in the setting of patients with MTS, the potential for memory decline is mitigated by the damage to the mesial structures already manifested both on imaging and in memory testing. Nevertheless, patients are cautioned about risk of some noticeable decline being possible for dominant-side SLAH. In the absence of preoperative verbal memory decline in the setting of dominant-side MTS, it is presumed that there exists

some contralateral mediation of verbal memory. In this setting, a strongly asymmetric Wada test showing ipsilaterally poor performance is reassuring, but risk of verbal memory decline with SLAH is not completely excluded and patients are thus counseled. Although our preliminary data suggest less impact on memory of SLAH compared with open resection, this conclusion awaits analysis of a larger group.

5. It has become our routine to offer dominant SLAH as the only first-line option for patients with MTS because of the significant potential for collateral damage and associated naming deficits associated with open resective approaches to the dominant side.[24] In those patients who do not achieve seizure freedom,

reablation is considered if delayed postoperative MRI shows persistent hippocampal or amygdalar remnants, but open resection may be considered as well.

Patients Without Mesial Temporal Sclerosis

Patients with MTLE without MTS may be at higher risk for failure after open temporal lobe surgery.[25] It is conceivable that a more focal procedure such as SLAH results in inferior rates of seizure freedom, but this is by no means certain, because in many cases, invasive recordings show onsets originating from the hippocampus in patients without MTS. Conversely, neurocognitive issues sway us to consider SLAH in patients with MTLE without MTS over open resection for 2 reasons: (1) patients without MTS are similarly (or more so) at risk for collateral damage from open procedures than are patients with MTS; and (2) memory is generally more preserved in patients without MTS; selective ablation of the amygdalohippocampal complex (relatively preserving entorhinal/parahippocampal cortex) is certainly not more deleterious to memory, and may be less so, compared with open resection. However, the seizure and neurocognitive outcomes in these groups remain to be determined. In our initial series, only 1 of 4 patients without MTS maintained seizure freedom for 6 months[10] and 2 years (R. Gross, J. Willie, unpublished observations, 2015). However, 1 of the patients who is not seizure free has a reduction in seizures greater than 85% and although 9 seizures localized unilaterally during preoperative LTVM, post-SLAH LTVM captured a contralateral seizure only. Another patient became seizure free for greater than 12 months after repeat SLAH targeting residual amygdalohippocampal tissue. Thus, this small sample size may underestimate the effectiveness of SLAH on the operated side even in patients without MTS.

Our present approach, therefore, involves offering SLAH to patients without MTS with onsets on the nondominant side in whom loss of visual memory function has been considered less consequential. However, because emerging data suggest underappreciation for at-risk temporal lobe functions (eg, recognition of familiar faces, landmarks, and animals; theory of mind and other more subtle aspects of social processing), we do discuss potential at-risk functions with our patients.[5,24,26,27] If a patient desires the most expeditious pathway to seizure freedom, we perform nondominant open resection if desired. If seizure freedom is not obtained after SLAH, repeat ablation or open resection is offered; LTVM is repeated only if there is a change of semiology or if there is a significant decrease in seizure frequency, suggesting the possibility that unrecognized contralateral seizures may account for the recurrence. On the other hand, we do not offer SLAH as a first-line measure to dominant onset patients without MTS unless there has already been significant loss of verbal memory, because such patients are at significant risk to memory in the setting of possible decreased chance of benefit; such patients are considered for neuromodulation. In the setting of dominant onset patients without MTS with more than mild verbal memory decline, and for patients who do not want neuromodulation and are willing to assume the risk of memory dysfunction on intensive preoperative counseling, we do offer SLAH and do not offer resection because of the risk to naming function of the latter. Open resection is offered only as a salvage measure if SLAH is not effective. One patient without MTS in our initial report (hippocampal T2 signal changes only) did not become seizure free with repeat ablation but did with subsequent ATL, whereas a more recent patient did not become seizure free after open SAH after failed SLAH. Such patients remain challenging. Routinely performing invasive monitoring with depth electrodes may be advisable in the evaluation for SLAH in patients without MTS. In our more extended series, 3 of 4 patients without MTS that localized to the hippocampus with depth electrodes have become seizure free (R. Gross, J. Willie, unpublished observations, 2015).

STEREOTACTIC LASER AMYGDALOHIPPOCAMPECTOMY: PROCEDURE
Stereotactic Planning

Stereotactic planning may be performed on any navigation workstation and can be performed ahead of time. A volumetric T1-weighted sequence with gadolinium contrast enhancement is necessary and can be supplemented with a T2 volumetric series.

- Choose an initial target point in the center of the pes hippocampus, that is, dentate gyrus
- Choose entry point in center of hippocampus at coronal level between the lateral mesencephalic sulcus and the tectal plate
- Extend the entry point to the skull; adjust the trajectory to:
  - Avoid cerebral veins and deep arterial branches
  - Avoid the ventricle (if possible); this usually involves an approach inferior to the occipital horn of the ventricle
  - Avoid the choroid plexus (if possible)

○ Keep the trajectory in the center of the hippocampus (dorsoventrally and mediolaterally)
• Extend the target point along the existing trajectory to just anterior to the amygdala

Stereotactic Insertion of Laser Fiber Assembly

Several techniques are available to insert the laser fiber assembly; our experience has been with the Visualase system (Medtronic, Louisville, CO) (**Fig. 3**). Any stereotactic approach may be used that maximizes stereotactic accuracy, including frame-based systems, frameless systems, or robot-assisted systems. However, a high level of accuracy is required because of the need to be centered within the hippocampus (coronally) and the constraints imposed by the need for accuracy all along the longitudinal trajectory.

The laser fiber assembly can be inserted through a stereotactically implanted anchor bolt in the operating room (OR) using a frame or frameless system (see **Fig. 3**). In this implementation, the following steps are taken:

• Insertion through anchor bolt in OR
  ○ Affix stereotactic frame. We perform this procedure under general anesthesia because it is unwise to perform procedures in awake epileptic patients unless necessary. This strategy avoids needing to intubate a patient with the frame in place; this could also be done with laryngeal mask anesthesia.

  ○ Imaging. Obtain volumetric contrast-enhanced MRI or contrast-enhanced CT merged with historical MRI.
  ○ Plan trajectory. As described earlier.
  ○ Positioning. Position supine with head flexed and maximally elevated (near sitting position) and anchor frame to table base unit. Minimal hair clipping followed by preparation and draping.
  ○ Stereotactic twist drill craniostomy. Use minimal stab incision.
  ○ Radiological control. Align C-arm fluoroscopy or intraoperative CT scanner.
  ○ Insert anchor bolt. Insert rod through frame bushing and then through the anchor bolt under fluoroscopic or CT control to make sure rod, and thus the anchor bolt, accurately achieves stereotactic target.
  ○ Insert cooling cannula. Remove rod and insert cooling cannula with inner stylet under guidance.
  ○ Insert fiber optic with diffusor tip. Remove stylet and insert optical fiber and secure. We use a 10-mm diffuser tip.
  ○ Remove frame arc but leave base ring in place.
  ○ Transport to the MRI suite. Patient positioned supine on the table with head turned to protect the laser assembly.
  ○ Confirm cannula accuracy and obtain scan planes for temperature mapping. If cannula is not accurately placed, the patient must be returned to the OR for repositioning.

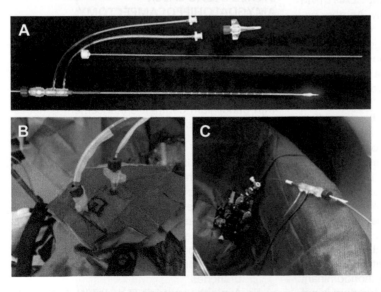

Fig. 3. Hardware components for SLAH using Visualase laser thermal therapy system using different stereotactic methods. (*A*) Fifteen-Watt 980-nm diode laser energy is directed along a 400-μm core silica optical fiber that terminates in a circumferential diffusing tip (*red*). This fiber optic is housed within a 1.65-mmdiameter saline-cooled polycarbonate cooling cannula (*bottom*). A threaded plastic bone anchor (*top right*) and stiffening stylet (*middle*) are used to stereotactically deliver the device to brain structures. (*B*) Stab incisions and 3.2-mm twist drill holes are made using a stereotactic headframe. Anchor bolts are threaded into twist holes under stereotactic control; Visualase laser applicators are passed through bolts, secured, and flagged with sterile adhesive strips. (*C*) Alternative direct real-time MRI-guided placement of Visualase laser applicator via an MRI guidance miniframe (SmartFrame, MRI Interventions, Irvine, CA) within an MRI suite. (*From* Willie JT, Tung JK, Gross RE. MRI-guided stereotactic laser ablation. Chapter 16. In: Golby AJ, editor. Image-guided neurosurgery. Boston: Academic Press; 2015. p. 380; with permission.)

Our alternative technique uses an MRI targeting platform in the MRI suite or intraoperative MR. This technique (1) allows the best three-dimensional radiologic targeting control and (2) avoids the need for transport of the patient during the procedure.

- Insertion using MRI targeting platform. We use the Clearpoint system (MRI Interventions, Irvine, CA) (see **Fig. 3**).
  - General anesthesia. General anesthesia is established in the MRI suite or OR.
  - Positioning. The patient is placed prone on the MRI table on bolsters and padded. The head is flexed and secured in skull pins. Clip hair, prepare, and drape. Affix a fiducial grid over the likely entry site, essentially 2 to 3 cm above the pinna, halfway between the pinna and the inion.[28]
  - Imaging. Volumetric T1 (eg, magnetization-prepared rapid gradient echo [MPRAGE]) with contrast.
  - Plan trajectory. As described earlier using Clearpoint workstation.
  - Affix scalp-mount Smartframe base and tower. This apparatus is centered over the entry point noted by the Clearpoint software and projected onto the skin using the fiducial grid.
  - Cannula alignment. This procedure is performed iteratively using serial slab MRI volumes guided by the software.
  - Twist drill craniotomy. Use minimal stab incision.
  - Insert ceramic stylet. Targeting accuracy is confirmed with a ceramic stylet with minimal image artifact inserted to target.
  - Insert cooling cannula. Replace ceramic with cooling cannula with stylet inserted to prescribed depth.
  - Insert optical fiber with diffusor tip. Remove stylet and insert optical fiber and secure. We use a 10-mm diffuser tip.
  - Confirm cannula accuracy and obtain scan planes for temperature mapping.

Laser Ablation with MRI Thermography

- Scan planes. Up to 3 scan planes (generally at least para-axially and parasagittally along the axis of the cannula) can be monitored with temperature mapping (T-maps) during the procedure. Additional planes increase the time between temperature updates. Although an additional coronal plane may be useful for monitoring the optic tract, new coronal scan planes would be necessary for each lesion along the longitudinal axis of the hippocampus.

- Attach optical fiber to laser power source; attach irrigation tubing. Confirm return flow of the irrigation before using laser.
- Choose safety monitoring points. The temperature at up to 6 points can be monitored. Typically 3 high points are chosen near the diffuser tip to ensure the temperature does not exceed 90°C to protect the tip. Three points are chosen on the brainstem, thalamus and optic tract to automatically turn off laser if temperature exceeds 45°C to 50°C.
- Low-power LITT. The laser is activated at 30% power (4.5 W) to verify the location of the diffuser tip; this can be translated in or out as needed. We begin the ablation at the anterior border of the amygdala.
- Create ablation. We typically create the first few overlapping ablations at 65% to 70% power (**Fig. 4**, Video 1). Each lesion is carried out until the pixels indicating the irreversible damage zone plateau, typically after 2 but no more than 3 minutes at a time. The cannula is then retracted 5 to 8 mm and overlapping ablations are serially performed as far back, but no further than, the tectal plate. For the posterior ablations, 60% power is sufficient and protects the optic radiation which is vulnerable here, as the diffuser tip may exit the hippocampus, and due to the narrowness of the lateral ventricle at this point.
- Postablation imaging. The immediate effects of the ablation are apparent on diffusion-weighted imaging, fluid-attenuated inversion recovery, T2, and gadolinium-enhanced T1 (eg, MPRAGE) imaging, the last of which shows the area of blood-brain barrier breakdown at the periphery of the lesion (see **Fig. 4**).
- Remove laser assembly, remove frame, single ligature of skin.

Postablation Management

- The patient is typically monitored for 1 night on the floor unit. No intensive care unit monitoring is required in the absence of a complication.
- Steroids are administered for 1 to 2 weeks. Transient headache is a common complaint after the procedure; this may be related to inflammogens released by the lesion coming in contact with the dura (eg, tentorial edge) but could also be related to local mass effect.
- Discharge on the day after surgery is typical.
- Antiepileptic medication is continued without change. We taper medications to some degree (eg, decreasing dosage[s] or eliminating a medication) if the patient remains seizure

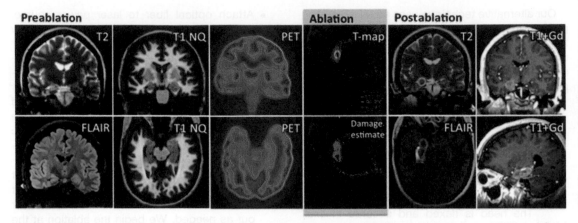

Fig. 4. Imaging associated with a case of SLAH for right MTS. Preablation diagnostic MRI (coronal T2 and fluid-attenuated inversion recovery [FLAIR], *first column*) show typical features of right hippocampal atrophy and mildly increased T2 and FLAIR intensity. Coronal and axial T1 with NeuroQuant (CorTechs Laboratory, San Diego, CA) analysis (*second column*) with colorized mesial temporal structures (*amygdala in blue, hippocampus in brown*) further exhibit right MTS. Coronal and axial FDG-PET images (*third column*) emphasize reduced hypometabolism of right mesial temporal structures. Visualase workstation screenshots during SLAH procedure (*fourth column*) show real-time axial MR gradient-based T-map during LITT in amygdala region (*above*) and combined irreversible damage estimate encompassing mesial temporal structures at time of procedure completion (*below*). Immediate postablation MR images show features after LITT including T2 (coronal) and FLAIR (axial) hypointense rings (*fifth column*), and peripheral contrast enhancement surrounding T1 hypointensity (coronal/sagittal gadolinium [Gd]-contrasted T1 images, *sixth column*).

free at 6 months but never discontinue medications completely until 2 years.

- Postoperative imaging beyond that acquired at the completion of the procedure is obtained only in the event of seizure recurrence.

TREATMENT RESISTANCE

Even in highly selected patients (eg, MTS), open resection is associated with a ~25% failure rate.[1] Some failed patients can be made seizure free by repeat surgery.[29] When patients are not seizure free after SLAH, we evaluate delayed MRI for remnant hippocampus/amygdala (although we never attempt full ablation of the most superior aspect of the amygdala because of continuity with basal ganglia and proximity to the optic tract). If remnants are present, these are targeted with a repeat procedure. Typically, remnant cortex is either mesial (subiculum) or lateral pes hippocampus or posterior body. Whereas entorhinal cortex (ECtx) and parahippocampal gyrus (PHG) are typically resected during open amygdalohippocampectomy, we do not target these in our initial procedure, and it remains uncertain whether PHG should be ablated during repeat procedures. Because the preservation of this region conceivably could account in part for better neurocognitive outcome after SLAH compared with open resection (particularly memory functions), we have generally elected not to target ECtx/PHG in our dominant-

sided reablations if there is persistent mesial temporal cortex that might account for failure but have performed more maximal ablations on the nondominant side. However, the precise neurocognitive consequences of repeated and more extensive ablations remain to be determined with more patients. Of 5 reablated patients with sufficient follow-up, 3 have become seizure free for 6 months or more. Conversely, only 1 of 3 patients who underwent ATL after SLAH became seizure free; 1 of these 3 patients had recurrent ipsilateral, contralateral, and psychogenic nonepileptic seizures, 1 had normal MRI, and the other had another possible ictal focus. This finding serves to emphasize that reasons for failure to control seizures may be assorted and multifactorial after both open resection and laser ablative surgery.

Our approach to recurrent seizures after SLAH is as follows (**Fig. 5**). Some seizures in the acute perioperative period (~6 weeks) do not necessarily indicate failure (winding-down phenomenon). However, persistent seizures after 2 months have invariably indicated failure and, in our experience, no such patient has experienced an extended seizure-free interval after this point. Thus, we evaluate patients for a follow-up procedure if recurrent seizures are present after 4 to 6 months. If seizures are of the same semiology as preoperatively, then further LTVM is not required before repeat SLAH. If there is persistent hippocampal or amygdalar tissue (uncus), then repeat ablation is offered. We

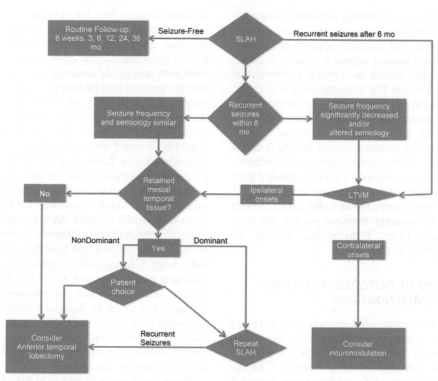

Fig. 5. Decision tree for further surgical treatment in non–seizure-free patients after SLAH. This is a guide to our decision making process in patients who are not seizure free after SLAH. Decision making may vary in a case-by-case manner depending on individual information and preferences.

offer open resection as an alternative in the case of seizure recurrence in patients after nondominant ablation. However, in the setting of dominant temporal lobe seizure recurrence, we avoid open resection if there is remnant tissue that may be ablated during a repeat procedure, because of the tangible risk of naming deficits with either dominant-sided ATL or SAH. Moreover, if we consider an open resection on the dominant side, we perform LTVM first to ensure that the recurrent seizures are still coming from the side of the previous ablation. Neurocognitive assessment and MRI are repeated before the patient undergoes a repeat procedure.

COMPLICATIONS

Complications (**Table 2**) from SLAH are related to the stereotactic approach, that is, brain penetration leading to hemorrhage and thermal effects on nearby structures. In 49 SLAH including 6 repeat procedures, we have experienced 2 tract hemorrhages: 1 small acute subdural hemorrhage and 1 temporo-occipital lobar hematoma associated with a transient visual field defect. Thermal injury can affect nearby visual pathways. One patient early on in the series experienced a subtotal

hemianopia most likely related to superior cannula deviation as seen on fluorography; there was no enhancement within the visual pathways to indicate thermal lesion. Two other patients

Table 2 Complications of stereotactic laser amygdalohippocampotomy	
Complication	**Incidence in 49 Procedures (6 Reoperations) (n) (%)**
Hemorrhage	2 (4.1)
Visual field deficit (total)	4 (8.2)
Transient (superior quadrantanopia)	1 (2.0)
Persistent	3 (6.1)
Homonymous heminanopia	1 (2.0)
Superior quadrantanopia	2 (4.1)
Cranial nerve deficit (transient)	2 (4.1)
CN3	1 (2.0)
CN4	1 (2.0)

experienced a non-disabling superior quadranta-nopia noted on clinical exam and field testing; however, we do not routinely perform postoperative visual field testing unless a patient is noted to have a field deficit on clinical confrontation testing. We believe the occurrence of a superior quadrantanopia can occur if a lesion is made too far posterolateral where the trajectory can encounter the optic radiation. Another location for thermal injury involves cranial nerves 3 and 4 if the lesion is made more medially near the tentorium. We have experienced 1 partial transient third nerve palsy with aggressive uncal ablation and 1 partial transient fourth nerve palsy with a repeat procedure to reablate remnant medial tissue at the subiculum/ECtx. Both partial deficits responded rapidly to steroids.

EVALUATION OF OUTCOME AND LONG-TERM RECOMMENDATIONS

Engel seizure classification scale is used to report outcome at 1 year after surgery. We have previously reported that 7 of our first 13 patients (54%) were seizure free at 6 months.[10] All remained seizure free at 1 year follow-up, except 1 patient having a single seizure only with rapid taper of lacosamide. All 7 remained seizure free at median 25 months (15–36 months) with the following exceptions: 1 patient had a single seizure with a dose of meperidine; 1 patient had 2 seizures with rapid taper of levatiracetam and concurrent hyponatremia; and 1 patient had 8 seizures over 4 months after discontinuing all of his seizure medications and binge drinking alcohol. In the last patient, control was regained with medications and he has been seizure free for an additional 12 months. Also, 1 patient from that initial series underwent repeat SLAH, resulting in seizure freedom for 1 year. Thus, the seizure-free rate at 12 months in this initial cohort has improved to 61.5%. Critically, 6 of 9 patients with MTS (67%) and 2 of 4 patients without MTS (50%) from the initial cohort are seizure free. The data from our larger series of 32 patients at 12 months follow-up are likewise consistent with these results (R. Gross, J. Willie, unpublished observations, 2015).

SUMMARY AND DISCUSSION

Open temporal lobe surgery for MTLE, having been performed in various forms for more than a half-century, is well established and effective. Class 1 evidence showed that 64% of operated patients became seizure free after ATL[30] and meta-analyses of numerous series of ATL and SAH[1] indicated that on average 75% of patients became seizure free for at least 1 year. Further, ATL and SAH are well-tolerated procedures that improve quality of life.[31] Nevertheless, we and others have shown that open resection is associated with previously unrecognized neurocognitive deficits beyond that related purely to the amygdalohippocampectomy,[5] as a result of collateral damage to the temporal lobe during the approach to the mesial temporal structures. This situation may be avoided with less invasive stereotactic procedures (see **Table 1**), but LITT has additional practical advantages over the alternatives.

We have shown in our initial series that SLAH is effective in eliminating seizures for follow-up periods of 15 to 36 months. As with open resection, superior results are obtained in patients with MTS (~70% seizure free thus far), rivaling the results from ATL and SAH. Patients failing to meet radiographic criteria for MTS are less likely to remain seizure free, but our experience with this group is too small to draw any conclusions, and these patients may go on to have additional procedures if indicated. However, we think it is important to continue to offer SLAH to patients without MTS for reasons discussed.

There are 2 areas in which SLAH offers distinct advantages over, and for these reasons may supplant, open resective surgery for MTLE as a first-line procedure for medication-resistant patients. First and foremost is the reduction of collateral damage to the lateral temporal structures, both gray and white matter, sparing patients from unnecessary neurocognitive deficits. We do not wish to underestimate the overriding importance of improvements in quality of life from seizure freedom after ATL/SAH. Nevertheless, neurocognitive deficits can remain bothersome and even disabling, especially in the dominant temporal lobe. Even when seizures are a distant memory, persistent deficits are not. Achieving seizure freedom and maximizing cognitive function by SLAH offers patients a distinct win/win. Second, as a so-called minimally invasive procedure, with a 1-stitch incision, SLAH is better tolerated and desirable to patients than even keyhole open resection, with no craniotomy and extracranial tissue injury. Postoperative intensive care admission/observation is obviated, and hospitalizations are brief. Many patients can return to work within days of SLAH.

Although it is clear to us that SLAH is the preferred treatment of patients with MTS and MTLE because of rates of seizure freedom comparable with open resection, the path remains less obvious for patients without MTS. Perhaps an isolated amygdalohippocampal ablation is too selective in the setting of uncertainty as to the onset region in these patients. However, in as much as the seizure network in this increasingly significant group of patients is poorly understood, a potentially superior procedure should not be withheld because of assumptions. Given the certain minimization of cognitive deficits, we believe it is important to explore the role of SLAH even in patients without MTS. It is for this reason that we also do not presuppose that such patients initially require more widespread ablations to include the PHG or the temporal pole. Perhaps we will learn that this factor is useful in the course of time, but to presuppose this may commit us to a larger surgery with greater deficits and preclude the opportunity to determine the minimum necessary substrate for achieving seizure freedom in various patient populations. The answer to the debate over "less is more" versus "more is more" is that "just right is more." The chance to iteratively enlarge the ablation/resection allows us to answer this question while we still have equipoise and while not subjecting patients to excessive risk. However, decisions are made in partnership with patients and caregivers. In particular cases, circumstances may be such (eg, limited social or economic resources) that we may have only 1 opportunity to intervene and provide the patient with a chance to be seizure free. If such patients can be identified prospectively ("we can always go back" is not always true), a resection rather than an ablation may be on balance more appropriate even on the dominant side.

The aforementioned considerations may have health care economic impacts. There clearly are savings from avoidance of intensive care unit observation as is routine after a craniotomy, and with nearly all patients being discharged on the morning after SLAH. Moreover, surgical time in the OR is decreased, and complications and discomfort related to craniotomy are eliminated. Conversely, there are increased technology expenses related to the disposable laser fiber assembly, the capital expense of the laser and computer workstation, and the opportunity cost of appropriating a diagnostic MRI scanner for interventional procedures that are more time consuming and potentially less profitable. The overall balance sheet with respect to these considerations is a topic we are pursuing.

SLAH has the potential to have even greater impact, related to its minimally invasive nature, by bringing more people with medication-resistant MTLE (and other forms of focal epilepsy) to surgical treatment. Epilepsy surgery use has lagged for decades, including for MTLE,[32] despite class 1 evidence supporting its effectiveness and safety since 2001.[30] This situation is related to reluctance by both patients and referring neurologists because of the invasiveness and side effects of open surgery. We have performed laser ablation on epileptic patients who have clearly stated that they would not consider open resection but were amenable to laser ablation. In this regard, comparison of seizure-free rates after SLAH to open resection captures only part of the picture; rather, for patients who accept this procedure but refuse open resection, the true comparator is best medical therapy, with its 8% chance of seizure freedom.[30] If one of the impacts of laser ablation is to bring more patients with epilepsy to surgery, with downstream benefits of decreasing medical complications (including sudden unexpected death from epilepsy) and increasing socioeconomic status, it will be a profound and persistent benefit to the community with epilepsy.

SUPPLEMENTARY DATA

Supplementary data related to this article can be found online at http://dx.doi.org/10.1016/j.nec. 2015.08.004.

REFERENCES

1. Josephson CB, Dykeman J, Fiest KM, et al. Systematic review and meta-analysis of standard vs selective temporal lobe epilepsy surgery. Neurology 2013;80(18):1669–76.
2. Mohammed HS, Kaufman CB, Limbrick DD, et al. Impact of epilepsy surgery on seizure control and quality of life: a 26-year follow-up study. Epilepsia 2012;53(4):712–20.
3. Helmstaedter C. Cognitive outcomes of different surgical approaches in temporal lobe epilepsy. Epileptic Disord 2013;15(3):221–39.
4. Baxendale S, Thompson PJ, Sander JW. Neuropsychological outcomes in epilepsy surgery patients with unilateral hippocampal sclerosis and good preoperative memory function. Epilepsia 2013;54(9): 131–4.
5. Drane DL, Loring DW, Voets NL, et al. Better object recognition and naming outcome with MRI-guided stereotactic laser amygdalohippocampotomy for temporal lobe epilepsy. Epilepsia 2015;56: 101–13.
6. Parent AG, Blume WT. Stereotactic amygdalohippocampotomy for the treatment of medial temporal lobe. Epilepsia 1999;40(10):1408–16.
7. Liscak R, Malikova H, Kalina M, et al. Stereotactic radiofrequency amygdalohippocampectomy in the treatment of mesial temporal lobe. Acta Neurochir (Wien) 2010;152(8):1291–8.
8. Bown SG. Phototherapy in tumors. World J Surg 1983;7(6):700–9.

9. Curry DJ, Gowda A, McNichols RJ, et al. MR-guided stereotactic laser ablation of epileptogenic foci in children. Epilepsy Behav 2012;24(4):408–14.

10. Willie JT, Laxpati NG, Drane DL, et al. Real-time magnetic resonance-guided stereotactic laser amygdalohippocampotomy for mesial temporal lobe epilepsy. Neurosurgery 2014;74(6):569–84 [discussion: 584–5].

11. Kwan P, Arzimanoglou A, Berg AT, et al. Definition of drug resistant epilepsy: consensus proposal by the ad hoc Task Force of the ILAE Commission on Therapeutic Strategies. Epilepsia 2010;51:1069–77.

12. Chabardes S, Kahane P, Minotti L, et al. The temporopolar cortex plays a pivotal role in temporal lobe seizures. Brain 2005;128(Pt 8):1818–31.

13. Drane DL. Neuropsychological evaluation of the epilepsy surgical candidate. In: Barr WB, Morrison C, editors. Handbook on the neuropsychology or epilepsy. New York: Springer; 2015. p. 87–122.

14. Loring DW, Meador KJ, Lee GP, et al. Amobarbital effects and lateralized brain function: the Wada test. New York: Springer-Verlag; 1992.

15. Kwan P, Brodie MJ. Refractory epilepsy: mechanisms and solutions. Expert Rev Neurother 2006; 6(3):397–406.

16. Mohanraj R, Brodie MJ. Diagnosing refractory epilepsy: response to sequential treatment schedules. Eur J Neurol 2006;13(3):277–82.

17. Kwan P, Brodie MJ. Early identification of refractory epilepsy. N Engl J Med 2000;342:314–9.

18. Schiller Y, Najjar Y. Quantifying the response to antiepileptic drugs: effect of past treatment history. Neurology 2008;70(1):54–65.

19. Engel J. Early surgical therapy for drug-resistant temporal lobe epilepsy. a randomized trial. JAMA 2012;307(9):922.

20. Laxpati NG, Kasoff WS, Gross RE. Deep brain stimulation for the treatment of epilepsy: circuits, targets, and trials. Neurotherapeutics 2014;11(3):508–26.

21. Wu C, Sharan AD. Neurostimulation for the treatment of epilepsy: a review of current surgical interventions. Neuromodulation 2013;16(1):10–24 [discussion: 24].

22. Bell ML, Rao S, So EL, et al. Epilepsy surgery outcomes in temporal lobe epilepsy with a normal MRI. Epilepsia 2009;50(9):2053–60.

23. Morrell MJ, RNS System in Epilepsy Study Group. Responsive cortical stimulation for the treatment of medically intractable partial epilepsy. Neurology 2011;77(13):1295–304.

24. Drane DL, Ojemann GA, Aylward E, et al. Category-specific naming and recognition deficits in temporal lobe epilepsy. Neuropsychologia 2008;46(5): 1242–55.

25. Wassenaar M, Leijten FS, Egberts TC, et al. Prognostic factors for medically intractable epilepsy: a systematic review. Epilepsy Res 2013;106(3): 301–10.

26. Crane J, Milner B. Do I know you? Face perception and memory in patients with selective amygdalo-hippocampectomy. Neuropsychologia 2002;40(5): 530–8.

27. Drane DL, Ojemann GA, Ojemann JG, et al. Category-specific recognition and naming deficits following resection of a right anterior temporal lobe tumor in a patient with atypical language lateralization. Cortex 2009;45(5):630–40.

28. Wu C, LaRiviere MJ, Laxpati N, et al. Extraventricular long-axis cannulation of the hippocampus: technical considerations. Neurosurgery 2014;10(Suppl 2): 325–32 [discussion: 332–3].

29. Germano IM, Poulin N, Olivier A. Reoperation for recurrent temporal lobe epilepsy. J Neurosurg 1994;81(1):31–6.

30. Wiebe S, Blume WT, Girvin JP, et al. A randomized, controlled trial of surgery for temporal-lobe epilepsy. N Engl J Med 2001;345:311–8.

31. Spencer SS, Berg AT, Vickrey BG, et al. Health-related quality of life over time since resective epilepsy surgery. Ann Neurol 2007;62(4):327–34.

32. Englot DJ, Ouyang D, Garcia PA, et al. Epilepsy surgery trends in the United States, 1990-2008. Neurology 2012;78(16):1200–6.

Minimally Invasive Neurosurgery for Epilepsy Using Stereotactic MRI Guidance

CrossMark

S. Kathleen Bandt, MD[a],*, Eric C. Leuthardt, MD[a,b,c]

KEYWORDS

- Medically refractory epilepsy • Laser ablation • Stereotactic guidance • Epilepsy surgery

KEY POINTS

- New, innovative, and minimally invasive, image-guided techniques for the surgical management of medically refractory epilepsy can be divided into thermoablative options and image-guided, robotic-assisted disconnective techniques.
- The most well described of these new minimally invasive options is laser thermoablation, which uses thermal energy delivered to a patient's unique seizure focus to locally destroy tissue under real-time magnetic resonance (MR) guidance.
- Larger series and longer follow-up periods will determine each individual option's long-term role in the surgical armamentarium for the treatment of medically refractory epilepsy but preliminary results seem promising.

INTRODUCTION

Approximately 1,000,000 Americans live with medically refractory epilepsy, and current surgical techniques address only a subset of this population's epileptic pathologies.[1] Although efficacious, there is an opportunity for improvement in the manner that the seizure focus is addressed. Surgical management typically involves an open craniotomy and either a removal of tissue or a disconnection procedure. As with all craniotomies, there are the attendant morbidities of bleeding, infection, postoperative pain, and wound complications. There has always a drive to reduce the invasiveness of these procedures to optimize the balance between the benefit of the surgery and the associated risks. Additionally, the risks of surgery may plan an adverse role in the perceptions of surgery as a therapeutic approach for epilepsy, thus potentially limiting the number of patients referred for surgical therapy despite level I evidence to the contrary.[2] These factors synergistically encourage the development of new and innovative treatment options that can diversify the surgical armamentarium for the treatment of medically refractory epilepsy. Several new minimally invasive treatment options have developed from this treatment gap and will hopefully contribute to its narrowing as they become more widely recognized and patient outcomes prove their long-term efficacy for the management of medically refractory epilepsy.

Commercial and/or Financial Conflicts of Interest: None.
[a] Department of Neurological Surgery, Washington University School of Medicine, Campus Box 8057, 660 South Euclid Avenue, St Louis, MO 63110, USA; [b] Department of Biomedical Engineering, Washington University, St Louis, MO 63110, USA; [c] Center for Innovation in Neuroscience and Technology, Washington University School of Medicine, St Louis, MO 63110, USA
* Corresponding author.
E-mail address: skbandt@gmail.com

PATIENT EVALUATION

Patients with medically refractory epilepsy referred to a tertiary-care epilepsy center for surgical consideration are reviewed by a multidisciplinary epilepsy team. This group typically includes the following members: (1) epilepsy neurologists who coordinate care and oversee video electroencephalogram (EEG) monitoring and interpretation; (2) specialized neuroradiologists trained in the interpretation of high-resolution MRI, typically including hippocampal volumetric analysis as well as PET and frequently single-photon emission CT (SPECT) imaging; (3) dedicated neuropsychologists who administer a battery of neuropsychological tests used to evaluate patients' cognitive function and predict cognitive outcomes across various surgical techniques based on preoperative performance; and (4) neurosurgeons with subspecialized training in the surgical treatment options for the management of medically refractory epilepsy. Patients who are reviewed by this multidisciplinary team may be found to warrant further work-up with intracranial monitoring, including either subdural and/or depth electrode placement if there is a discordance between seizure semiology, imaging, or EEG findings. Alternatively, if there is concordance across these various categories, patients are referred directly for surgical treatment of their medically refractory epilepsy.

SURGICAL TREATMENT OPTIONS

Historically, treatment options were divided into 2 categories: resective or disconnective. Resective treatment strategies included removal of the epileptogenic focus. Some of the most common surgical procedures include temporal lobectomy, selective amygdalohippocampectomy, and topectomy of the neocortical tissue, which was believed to be a patient's epileptogenic focus. Disconnective treatment strategies include disconnection of epileptogenic brain from nonepileptogenic brain by corpus callosotomy or hemispherotomy, both of which are typically reserved for palliative treatment of pediatric epilepsy. Additional accepted surgical treatment options for medically refractory epilepsy include neuromodulatory techniques, including vagal nerve stimulation and more recently responsive neurostimulation. Additional stereotactic MR-guided treatment options for the management of medically refractory epilepsy have also been recently introduced. These newer techniques are thermoablative in nature, such that rather than removing the tissue, the site is destroyed in situ.

Thermoablative Techniques

Multiple thermoablative treatment strategies have developed over the past 25 years and all rely on the basic principle of heating tissue to result in protein denaturation and tissue destruction. The energy source by which this thermoablative process occurs varies across the different techniques and includes laser, radiofrequency, and ultrasound-induced forms of thermal tissue destruction.

Laser thermoablation

Since its introduction to neurosurgery in 1990 and with an increasing presence since 2007, laser ablative techniques have been applied to the management of unresectable tumors,[3–7] mesial temporal lobe epilepsy,[8] neocortical dysplasia,[9] poststroke neocortical seizure foci,[10] periventricular nodular heterotopia,[11] and hypothalamic hamartomas,[12] among others. There are currently 2 commercially available devices used to carry out these ablative procedures. The first of these to receive Food and Drug Administration approval was the Visualase system in 2007 (Medtronic, Minneapolis, Minnesota) and more recently the NeuroBlate System in 2010 (Monteris Medical, Plymouth, Minnesota). Both systems offer stereotactic access to deep and superficial lesions and provide concentric laser ablation capabilities. Conformal laser ablation is additionally provided by the NeuroBlate System, which offers the option of a directionally oriented laser source to guide delivery of thermal energy for more irregularly shaped surgical targets.

Regardless of which system is used, the surgical technique includes the patient undergoing a preablation localizing MRI from which a volumetric target is selected for ablation. The thermal energy source is then placed under stereotactic guidance, allowing delivery of the thermoablative energy. Live intraprocedural repetitive measurements of a T1-weighted 2-D– fast low-angle shot (FLASH) sequence provide temporally sensitive thermometry measurements necessary to inform and control the energy delivered to create controlled and conformal lesions (**Fig. 1**). These lesions are verifiable with postablation diffusion-weighted MRI, evidence of hemorrhagic necrosis on T1-weighted imaging, and a new distribution of gadolinium enhancement (**Fig. 2**).

A review of the literature and the authors' experience include the following applications for laser ablation for the management of medically refractory epilepsy.

Mesial temporal lobe epilepsy Willie and colleagues[8] report the successful application of laser

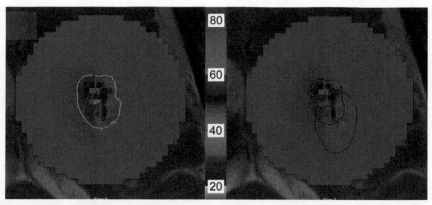

Fig. 1. Real-time heat map of thermal energy delivered under MR guidance.

thermoablation to mesial temporal lobe epilepsy with their report of 13 patients undergoing laser thermoablation of the amygdala, hippocampus, and parahippocampal gyrus. Seizure outcomes were nearly comparable to open resection of the mesial temporal structures with selective amygdalohippocampectomy, with 77% (10/13) of patients enjoying significant reduction of seizure burden (Engel class I–III) and 54% (7/13) free of disabling seizures (Engel class I). Mean mesial temporal lobe ablation volume averaging at 60% without an apparent dose-dependent relationship between ablation volume and seizure outcome, suggesting subtotal ablation can be associated with favorable seizure outcome.

Cortical dysplasias
Case 1 A 26 year-old woman with 8-year history of medically refractory epilepsy was found to have a right temporal cortical malformation, which corresponded with her EEG seizure onset and demonstrated hypometabolism on PET imaging (**Fig. 3**). This patient was offered either surgical resection or laser ablation and elected to proceed with laser ablation. She remains seizure-free 18 months postoperatively.

Case 2 Clarke and colleagues[9] report the successful laser thermoablation of a patient with bilateral occipital cortical dysplasias, highlighting the successful application of this technique to pathologies associated with eloquent cortex and well as the role of multifocal ablation in patients with multifocal seizure onset, which would previously have been considered not amenable to surgical resection.

Neocortical, magnetic resonance–negative focus A 57-year-old woman with a 42-year history

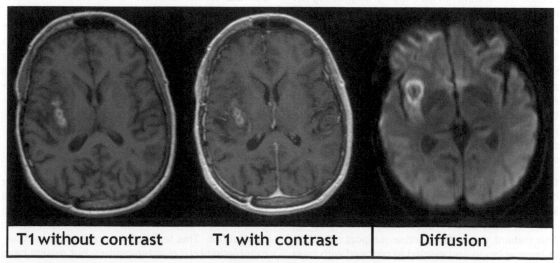

| T1 without contrast | T1 with contrast | Diffusion |

Fig. 2. Postablation T1-weighted sequences with (*middle*) and without (*left*) contrast and diffusion-weighted sequence demonstrating treatment effect (*right*).

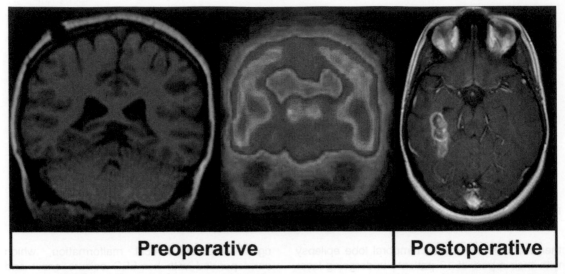

Fig. 3. Preoperative (*left*) and postoperative (*right*) MRI and PET images demonstrating hypometabolic left temporal cortical dysplasia and resulting postablation contrast enhancement (*middle*).

of medically refractory epilepsy after a motor vehicle collision at age 15 without definite loss of consciousness now with medically refractory epilepsy. Preoperative work-up, including ictal SPECT, identified an MR-negative right insular seizure focus. The patient underwent laser ablation of this seizure focus and remains seizure-free 6 months postoperatively, although she developed a mild left hemiparesis after surgery, which continues to improve with therapy services and does not limit her ability to ambulate.

Poststroke neocortical seizure focus A 53-year-old man presents with 10-year history of medically refractory epilepsy. Preoperative evaluation demonstrated discordance in his imaging, suggesting left insular hypometabolism on PET associated with a prior silent infarction and diffuse left hippocampal fluid-attenuated inversion recovery (FLAIR) hyperintensity on MRI (**Fig. 4**). For this reason, this patient underwent placement of left subtemporal strips and left insular depth electrodes for intracranial monitoring and seizure localization. Ultimately, the patient's left insular focus was identified with invasive physiology and he underwent subsequent conformal laser ablation of this insular focus. He remains seizure-free 4 years postoperatively.

Encephalocele A 51-year-old woman with 22-year history of medically refractory epilepsy had a basal left temporal encephalocele, which corresponded with her EEG seizure-onset localization (**Fig. 5**). This patient was offered either surgical resection or laser ablation and elected to proceed with laser ablation. She remains seizure-free 2 years postoperatively.

Periventricular nodular heterotopia Esquenazi and colleagues[11] report the successful application of laser thermoablation to medically refractory epilepsy associated with periventricular nodular heterotopia. Historically, this disorder of neuronal migration, which is frequently associated with medically refractory epilepsy, has not been included in the surgically treatable category of drug-resistant epilepsy. MR-guided laser thermoablation will potentially expand this definition by accessing deep-seated lesions that typically are not considered amenable to open surgical resection.

Hypothalamic hamartoma Curry and colleagues[12] report the successful laser thermoablation of hypothalamic hamartomas in 2 children without significant associated hypothalamic dysfunction. Historically, hypothalamic hamartomas have been challenging to treat due to their association with medically refractory epilepsy and the associated risks of hypothalamic dysfunction with open microsurgical resection. Stereotactic laser thermoablation may represent a promising new treatment option for these challenging lesions.

Radiofrequency thermoablation
Radiofrequency thermoablation involves the stereotactic placement of a radiofrequency emitter source, which administers current at frequencies greater than 250 kHz to heat surrounding tissues to the point of protein denaturation and tissue destruction. This technology predates laser thermoablation by a quarter-century but results have been mixed and reporting of outcomes confined to small case series over time.[13–15] This has

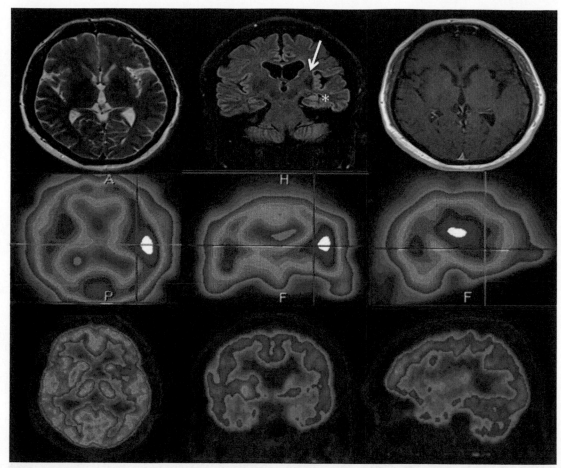

Fig. 4. Preoperative imaging demonstrating left hippocampal hyperintensity (*asterisk*) and left insular hypointensity (*arrow*) on FLAIR sequence (*top row, middle*). Ictal SPECT identifies left insular hyperperfusion (*middle row*) and PET suggests left insular hypometabolism (*bottom row*). This discordance led to intracranial monitoring, which identified a left insular seizure focus.

contributed to a slow adoption of this technology, although some reports suggest favorable long-term outcomes. This technology has been used primarily for the treatment of medically refractory mesial temporal lobe epilepsy and hypothalamic hamartomas, although significant transient hypothalamic dysfunction has been reported with its application to hypothalamic hamartomas.[13]

Focused ultrasound thermoablation

Focused ultrasound thermoablation uses transcranial array of ultrasonic emitter sources, allowing differential frequency delivery ranging from 230 to 1000 kHz to stereotactically target structures for thermocoagulation.[16] This technology remains largely experimental at this point but represents an innovative, potentially noninvasive treatment modality for medically refractory epilepsy.

Magnetic Resonance–Guided, Robot-Assisted Disconnective Techniques

In addition to the different varieties of thermoablative techniques at the epilepsy surgeon's disposal, there is an alternative, minimally invasive technique that represents an update to the classic disconnective surgical options. This is the use of an MR-guided laser source to perform disconnection of either periharmartomatous tissue or the corpus callosum. The thulium laser technology capitalizes on stereotactic guidance and robotic assistance simultaneously. Currently, its application hypothalamic hamartoma has been described[17] but conceivably, it could be applied to standard disconnective surgical procedures today, including corpus callosotomy and/or hemispherotomy. There have also been recent demonstrations of minimally invasive open procedures in which flexible CO_2

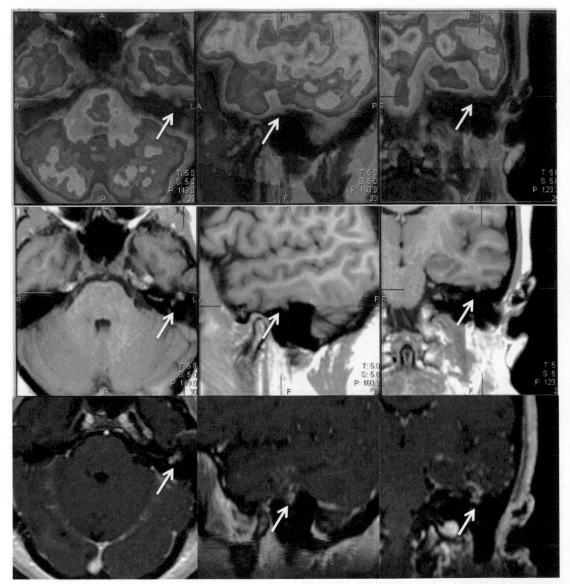

Fig. 5. Preoperative PET and MRI demonstrating patient's hypometabolic right basal temporal encephalocele. Postoperative MRI demonstrating postablation contrast enhancement. Arrows identifies encephalocele.

lasers have used for corpus callosotomies.[18] Additionally, these technologies may represent new disconnective modalities for adjunctive transective procedures along the epilepsy network, which have been described as associated with seizure propagation.[19]

COMPLICATIONS

Despite the minimally invasive nature of these surgical procedures, they are not without the risks associated with surgery. The minimally invasive feature of these different surgical offerings do

provide the unique benefit of shorter length of both ICU stay and overall hospital stay compared with their open surgical counterparts.[8] They may also be associated with shorter return to work times for patients who are gainfully employed at the time of their surgical procedure. Known complications associated with all surgery for epilepsy are the risks of postoperative bleeding, including surgical site hematoma formation. One notable risk given the small surgical exposure is the possibility of postoperative subdural hematoma formation associated with dural penetration in proximity to a cortical vessel, which would otherwise be controlled under direct visualization in open surgical technique. Willie and colleagues[8] report a single small acute subdural hematoma in their case series of laser thermoablation for mesial temporal lobe epilepsy. Given that most of these procedures are performed under real-time MR guidance, if a hematoma were to develop within the surgical site during the procedure, it would likely be identified intraoperatively and, therefore, could be managed at the time of its occurrence.

Additionally, the risks associated with temporal lobe surgery, including postoperative visual field deficits and language and/or memory deficits, would persist for these minimally invasive approaches as they would for open surgical techniques. That said, Drane and colleagues[20] note improved cognitive outcomes than what otherwise would be expected in their series of using thermoablation of the mesial temporal lobe structures. Likewise, surgery for hypothalamic hamartomas has been associated with the development of postoperative hypothalamic dysfunction. Although this risk remains, reports suggest the permanence of this dysfunction may be minimized by using minimally invasive techniques compared with open surgical techniques.[13]

EVALUATION OF OUTCOME AND LONG-TERM RECOMMENDATIONS

These innovative treatment options and their application to the surgical management of medically refractory epilepsy is too new to have enough data to make long-term assessments of efficacy and patient satisfaction. Each of these modalities has been described in the treatment of medically refractory epilepsy only in small case series and case report format and is only theoretic in the case of focused ultrasound ablation. Larger series and longer follow-up periods will determine each option's long-term role in the surgical armamentarium for the treatment of medically refractory epilepsy but preliminary results seem promising.

SUMMARY

In addition to the time-honored, proved techniques of open surgery for the management of medically refractory epilepsy, there are many new, innovative, minimally invasive options that may prove to fundamentally change the field of epilepsy surgery or may simply diversify a field of equally robust treatment options. They represent an emerging reality in the field of epilepsy surgery and offer exciting frontiers for further consideration and investigation.

To define appropriate care algorithms, more robust evidence is needed going forward. Specific questions that likely require multicenter randomized controlled trials will be the comparative efficacy of open surgical treatment versus minimally invasive approaches. Also, for those diagnoses (eg, deep lesions and multifocal onset) where open surgery is generally not considered an option, more exhaustive prospective registries likely will be needed to define the clinical benefit and risks of these emerging treatments as formal comparison to best medical management. These open questions and emerging capabilities set the stage for an exciting future of development within the field of epilepsy surgery.

REFERENCES

1. Hauser WA. The natural history of drug resistant epilepsy: epidemiologic considerations. Epilepsy Res Suppl 1992;5:25–8.
2. Wiebe S, Blume WT, Girvin JP, et al. A randomized, controlled trial of surgery for temporal-lobe epilepsy. N Engl J Med 2001;345(5):311–8.
3. Bettag M, Ulrich F, Schober R, et al. Stereotactic laser therapy in cerebral gliomas. Acta Neurochir Suppl (Wien) 1991;52:81–3.
4. Kahn T, Bettag M, Ulrich F, et al. MRI-guided laser-induced interstitial thermotherapy of cerebral neoplasms. J Comput Assist Tomogr 1994;18(4):519–32.
5. Carpentier A, Chauvet D, Reina V, et al. MR-guided laser-induced thermal therapy (LITT) for recurrent glioblastomas. Lasers Surg Med 2012;44(5):361–8.
6. Mohammadi AM, Hawasli AH, Rodriguez A, et al. The role of laser interstitial thermal therapy in enhancing progression-free survival of difficult-to-access high-grade gliomas: a multicenter study. Cancer Med 2014;3(4):971–9.
7. Hawasli AH, Kim AH, Dunn GP, et al. Stereotactic laser ablation of high-grade gliomas. Neurosurg Focus 2014;37(6):E1.
8. Willie JT, Laxpati NG, Drane DL, et al. Real-time magnetic resonance-guided stereotactic laser amygdalohippocampotomy for mesial temporal lobe epilepsy. Neurosurgery 2014;74(6):569–84 [discussion: 584–5].
9. Clarke DF, Tindall K, Lee M, et al. Bilateral occipital dysplasia, seizure identification, and ablation: a novel surgical technique. Epileptic Disord 2014;16(2):238–43.
10. Hawasli AH, Bandt SK, Hogan RE, et al. Laser ablation as treatment strategy for medically refractory dominant insular epilepsy: therapeutic and functional considerations. Stereotact Funct Neurosurg 2014;92(6):397–404.

11. Esquenazi Y, Kalamangalam GP, Slater JD, et al. Stereotactic laser ablation of epileptogenic periventricular nodular heterotopia. Epilepsy Res 2014; 108(3):547–54.

12. Curry DJ, Gowda A, McNichols RJ, et al. MR-guided stereotactic laser ablation of epileptogenic foci in children. Epilepsy Behav 2012;24(4):408–14.

13. Kameyama S, Murakami H, Masuda H, et al. Minimally invasive magnetic resonance imaging-guided stereotactic radiofrequency thermocoagulation for epileptogenic hypothalamic hamartomas. Neurosurgery 2009;65(3):438–49 [discussion: 449].

14. Patil AA, Andrews R, Torkelson R. Stereotactic volumetric radiofrequency lesioning of intracranial structures for control of intractable seizures. Stereotact Funct Neurosurg 1995;64(3):123–33.

15. Liscak R, Malikova H, Kalina M, et al. Stereotactic radiofrequency amygdalohippocampectomy in the treatment of mesial temporal lobe epilepsy. Acta Neurochir (Wien) 2010;152(8):1291–8.

16. Monteith S, Sheehan J, Medel R, et al. Potential intracranial applications of magnetic resonance-guided focused ultrasound surgery. J Neurosurg 2013;118(2):215–21.

17. Calisto A, Dorfmüller G, Fohlen M, et al. Endoscopic disconnection of hypothalamic hamartomas: safety and feasibility of robot-assisted, thulium laser-based procedures. J Neurosurg Pediatr 2014;14(6):563–72.

18. Choudhri O, Lober RM, Camara-Quintana J, et al. Carbon dioxide laser for corpus callosotomy in the pediatric population. J Neurosurg Pediatr 2015; 15(3):321–7.

19. Bandt SK, Bundy DT, Hawasli AH, et al. The role of resting state networks in focal neocortical seizures. PLoS One 2014;9(9):e107401.

20. Drane DL, Loring DW, Voets NL, et al. Better object recognition and naming outcome with MRI-guided stereotactic laser amygdalohippocampotomy for temporal lobe epilepsy. Epilepsia 2015;56(1):101–13.

Stereotactic Laser Ablation for Hypothalamic Hamartoma

John D. Rolston, MD, PhD, Edward F. Chang, MD*

KEYWORDS

- Gelastic seizures • Refractory epilepsy • Hypothalamic hamartoma • Laser • Ablation
- Technical approach

KEY POINTS

- Stereotactic laser ablation (SLA) is a minimally invasive approach to the treatment of medication-resistant epilepsy that accomplishes ablation of the seizure focus with real-time magnetic resonance thermal mapping.
- Rates of seizure freedom in early series suggest that SLA approaches and perhaps surpasses the effectiveness of open resection.
- SLA minimizes the neurocognitive and endocrine adverse effects of open surgery.
- Secondary benefits of SLA include decreased length of stay, elimination of intensive care unit stay, reduced procedure-related discomfort, and improved access to surgical treatment for patients less likely to consider an open resective procedure.

INTRODUCTION

Hypothalamic hamartomas (HHs) are non-neoplastic developmental malformations centered around the tuber cinereum. They are associated with medically refractory epilepsy, developmental delays, and often precocious puberty (up to 40% of cases).[1] Pathologically, HHs are characterized by disorganized glioneuronal tissue, and can be readily divided into 2 types: sessile and pedunculated,[2] with many other specific classifications also proposed, such as that by Delalande and Fohlen,[3] which divides HHs into type I (within the tuber cinereum, usually eccentric to one side), type II (intraventricular), type III (mixed), and type IV (giant, >2 cm in diameter).

Gelastic seizures (GSs) are the first and most specific type of seizure experienced by patients with HHs. GSs vary from feeling a mild "pressure to laugh," to uncontrollable outbursts of laughter, during which consciousness is usually maintained.

These mechanical bursts of laughter are not experienced as mirthful, and are often associated with concomitant autonomic signs, such as mydriasis and facial flushing.[1]

Up to 75% of patients with GSs go on to develop other types of intractable seizures, ranging from partial motor to generalized tonic-clonic. This secondary epileptogenesis is presumed due to the HH and resultant GSs, akin to a kindling effect.[4,5] This same process also appears to drive the resultant encephalopathy responsible for behavioral, cognitive, and psychiatric impairments in patients with HH. Importantly, surgical ablation of the HH can reverse this encephalopathy, reducing the frequency of seizures and improving cognitive and behavioral functioning.[6–8]

Many techniques have been used to remove and disconnect HHs, including open surgery, endoscopic approaches, stereotactic radiofrequency (RF) ablation, and stereotactic radiosurgery. Open

Disclosures: None.
Department of Neurological Surgery, University of California, San Francisco, 505 Parnassus Ave., M779, San Francisco, CA 94143, USA
* Corresponding author.
E-mail address: Edward.Chang@ucsf.edu

Neurosurg Clin N Am 27 (2016) 59–67
http://dx.doi.org/10.1016/j.nec.2015.08.007
1042-3680/16/$ – see front matter © 2016 Elsevier Inc. All rights reserved.

surgical approaches include transcallosal (primarily for Delalande types II, III, and IV) and skull base approaches, such as orbitozygomatic or pterional craniotomies (primarily for types I, III, and IV).[9] These procedures lead to seizure freedom in approximately 50% of patients, but have a high rate of complications, including transient memory disturbances in roughly half of the transcallosal patients and sporadic diabetes insipidus, poikilothermia, visual field deficits, and hemiparesis in the skull base patients.[9,10]

Complete endoscopic resection of HHs is technically difficult: for example, Rekate and colleagues[11] report a series of 44 patients, of whom they achieved total resection in just 14 (32%). The complication rate in this series was 25%, although most were transient.[11] When resection fails, disconnection of the HH using endoscopic surgery is another option, and again leads to a roughly 50% rate of seizure freedom.[12,13]

MRI-guided stereotactic RF ablation, although a more recent development, is a technically less-invasive technique than open surgery, with rates of seizure freedom approaching 75%,[14] although it nevertheless harbors similar complications to open surgical procedures (memory loss, brainstem infarctions, and cranial nerve palsies).[15]

Several methods of stereotactic radiosurgery have been used for HHs. Gamma Knife radiosurgery has been the most studied modality, and showed a 37% seizure freedom rate without permanent complications in the largest series to date (27 patients with adequate follow-up).[16] Linear accelerators have shown less success, with 2 small reports showing no improvement,[17,18]

and 1 showing seizure freedom in 2 of 3 patients.[19] All radiosurgery modalities take a substantial time period for effects to manifest, usually on the course of 1 to 2 years.

A more recent approach to the treatment of HHs is MRI-guided laser ablation. There has been only one study published to date using laser ablation, but the results were favorable, with 86% of 14 patients achieving complete seizure freedom, and an absence of any permanent side effects (**Table 1**).[20]

Laser Interstitial Thermal Therapy

During laser interstitial thermal therapy (LITT), laser light is delivered fiberoptically into tissue (interstitial) via a stereotactic approach. Unlike RF ablation, LITT uses photonic energy for thermocoagulation. Several critical advances have made modern LITT platforms into elegant and powerful neurosurgical tools (**Box 1**). The most critical advance is the ability to use MRI thermometry to measure not only the temperature at the device tip (the only temperature monitored in RF ablation), but also the temperature of tissue any distance from the tip during heating, thus providing near real-time confirmation of the ablation zone relative to off-target structures.

The photonic mechanism of heating is different from RF ablation, but the effects of temperature on tissue are the same. Although, again, thermometry allows monitoring of distal effects of heating, as compared with only tip measurements with radiofrequency probes. This technology allows protection of off-target tissue at risk in a way that is

Table 1
Approaches to hypothalamic hamartoma

Technique	Pros	Cons
Open surgery • Endoscopic • Craniotomy	Direct visualization	• High risk for morbidity ○ Memory impairments ○ Endocrine dysfunction ○ General surgical (eg, infection, stroke)
Stereotactic radiosurgery (SRS)	Noninvasive	• Delayed benefit after initial increase in seizures (risk of sudden unexpected death in epilepsy with continued seizures) • Potential radiation injury, dose limitations • High cost
Laser interstitial thermal therapy (LITT)	Minimal collateral damage Immediate benefit Near real-time MR thermography guides therapy and confirms ablation zone	• High cost/disposables • Must be cleared for MRI (excluding patients with implantable devices)

Box 1
Laser interstitial thermal therapy

- Optical fiber with diffusing tip (10 or 3 mm)
- Cooling cannula to control thermal spread within tissue and protect device tip
- 984-nm diode laser causes rapid heating of water within tissue
- Magnetic resonance thermography reads temperature change in all voxels
- 6 safety points to automatically shut off laser if temperature limits exceeded
- Irreversible damage zone estimate at each voxel based on Arrhenius equation

---

not possible with standard use of RF ablation. At present, 2 LITT devices are available in the United States that offer overlapping but distinctive features. Our study has used only the Visualase (Medtronic, Minneapolis, MN; **Fig. 1**).

CASE EXAMPLES
Case 1

A 28-year-old man with an HH presented to us for continued refractory seizures, despite Gamma Knife surgery when he was 20 years old (**Fig. 2**). His seizures included classic GSs, but also intermittent generalized tonic-clonic seizures, which occurred several times per year. Because of his continued refractory seizures, laser ablation was offered and the patient and family requested that surgery proceed.

In the computed tomography (CT) suite, the patient was placed under general anesthesia and intubated. A Leksell head frame was placed and a stereotactic head CT obtained. This CT was coregistered with a preoperative MRI. A trajectory was planned with an entry point at the right frontal

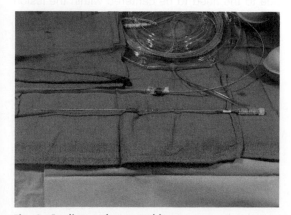

Fig. 1. Cooling catheter and laser.

convexity, along the coronal suture. Sulci and ventricles were avoided (**Fig. 3**).

The patient was taken to the operating room (OR) and placed in a semisitting position. After routine skin preparation and draping, the Leksell frame was applied and a twist-drill opening made in the skull. The Visualase sheath was passed to the target and secured with a bolt (**Fig. 4**). Intraoperative fluoroscopy was used to confirm this trajectory (**Fig. 5**). The patient was then removed from the frame and taken to the intraoperative MRI suite.

MRI was used to confirm the location of the cannula (**Fig. 6**). Two lesions were created, with temperature stops in the fornix and thalamus. Posttreatment MRI showed contrast enhancement of the lesion (see **Fig. 6**E, F). The patient then returned to the OR where the probe was removed and his wound closed.

Postoperatively, the patient continued to be seizure free at his most recent 5-month follow-up visit. He had transient hyperphagia and amnesia after the ablation, both of which were completely resolved at follow-up.

Case 2

The second case was a 20-year-old man with a right inferior HH, who had undergone 2 previous Gamma Knife treatments (once when 14, then again when 17) with only brief remissions of his seizures after both sessions (**Fig. 7**A, B). He suffered from complex partial seizures, which occurred several times monthly. He had no GSs. Given his continued intractable seizures despite medications and radiosurgery, he was presented with the option of MRI-guided laser ablation, and requested that surgery proceed.

As in case 1, general anesthesia was induced and the patient was intubated before a localizing CT. This was merged with a preoperative MRI and a trajectory was planned from the left. The sheath was placed in the OR, as in case 1, and the patient was then transferred to the MRI suite (**Fig. 7**C).

MRI was used to confirm the location of the laser probe (**Fig. 7**D). One lesion was made with the laser, and temperature stops were used in the cistern, optic nerve, and normal hypothalamus. Posttreatment MRI showed contrast enhancement of the lesion and sparing of the normal tissue.

The patient then returned to the OR where the Visualase sheath was removed and the burr hole closed.

At his most recent 7-month follow-up, the patient remains completely seizure free, although

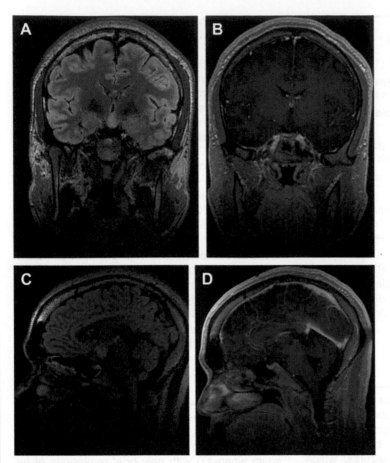

Fig. 2. Preoperative MRI of case 1. (*A*) Coronal FLAIR showing the HH, eccentric to the left. (*B*) Coronal contrast-enhanced T1-weighted image showing hypointense lesion in the hypothalamus. (*C*) Sagittal FLAIR again showing the hyperintense HH. (*D*) Contrast-enhanced sagittal image.

continues to have some auras, which last a few seconds and are not experienced as disabling. He has reduced his antiepileptic medications. There were no complications.

STEREOTACTIC LASER ABLATION: PROCEDURE
Stereotactic Planning

Stereotactic planning may be performed on any navigation workstation and can be performed ahead of time. A volumetric T1-weighted sequence with gadolinium enhancement is necessary, and can be supplemented with a T2-weighted volumetric series.

With the planning software, first choose an initial target point directly within the center of the tumor. Next, choose an entry point in the right or left frontal convexity, typically at or anterior to the coronal suture. Adjust this trajectory to avoid sulci, cerebral veins, arterial branches, and ventricles. When the trajectory is satisfactory, extend the depth to the bottom or most distal point of the tumor, although still on the same trajectory.

Stereotactic Insertion of Laser Fiber Assembly

Several techniques are available to insert the laser fiber assembly, which in our experience has been the Visualase system (see **Fig. 1**). Any stereotactic approach may be used that maximizes stereotactic accuracy, including frame-based systems, frameless systems, or robot-assisted systems. However, a high level of accuracy is required due to the need to be centered within the lesion and the constraints imposed by the need for accuracy all along the longitudinal trajectory (see **Fig. 3**).

The laser fiber assembly can be inserted through a stereotactically implanted anchor bolt in the OR using a frame or frameless system. This implementation uses the following steps. First, affix the stereotactic frame (the Leksell frame at our institution; see **Fig. 4**). We perform this under general anesthesia because it is unwise to perform procedures in awake epileptic patients unless necessary. This avoids needing to intubate a patient with the frame in place. This also could be done with laryngeal mask anesthesia.

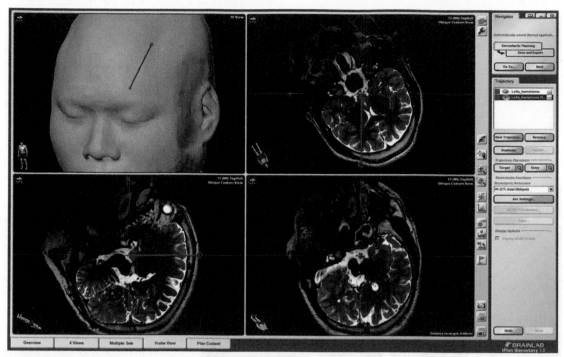

Fig. 3. Trajectory planning for case 1.

Next, obtain volumetric contrast-enhanced MRI or contrast-enhanced CT coregistered with the preoperative MRI. Trajectory planning then proceeds as previously described if not already done. In the OR, the patient should be positioned supine with his or her head flexed and maximally elevated (semisitting position) and the frame should be anchored to the operating table. The frame should be used to map out the entry point. Then, a minimal head shave is done, followed by preparation and draping of the patient.

Using a minimal stab incision, a twist-drill craniostomy is made at the insertion site (mapped out with the stereotactic frame). Intraoperative CT or fluoroscopy is then aligned with the patient. Next, the Visualase rod is inserted through the frame bushing and then through the anchor bolt under fluoroscopic or CT control. The imaging

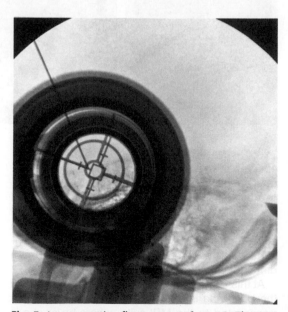

Fig. 5. Intraoperative fluoroscopy of case 1. The cannula is positioned just above arc center in the Leksell frame.

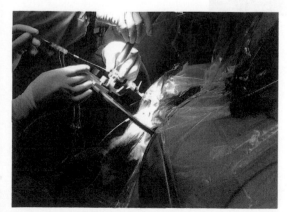

Fig. 4. Stereotactic placement of laser. Fluoroscopy guidance is used to confirm the cannula trajectory.

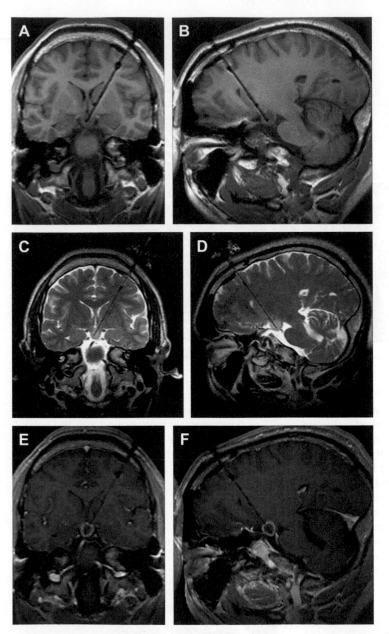

Fig. 6. Intraoperative MRI of case 1. (*A*, *B*) Coronal and sagittal T1-weighted images showing the cannula within the HH. (*C*, *D*) Coronal and sagittal T2-weighted images showing the cannula well-positioned. (*E*, *F*) Postoperative contrast-enhanced coronal and sagittal images showing ring-enhancement of the lesion.

ensures the rod, and thus the anchor bolt, accurately achieves its stereotactic target.

After the anchor is inserted, the rod is removed and replaced with the cooling cannula and inner stylet, again using imaging guidance. The stylet is then removed and the optical fiber is inserted and secured. We use a 3-mm or 10-mm diffuser tip.

At this stage, the frame arc is removed, although the base ring is left in place. The patient is then transported to the MRI suite, where he or she is positioned supine on the MRI table with the head turned to protect the laser assembly.

MRI is then used to confirm cannula accuracy and obtain scan planes for temperature mapping. If the cannula is misplaced, the patient must return to the OR for repositioning.

Laser Ablation with MRI Thermography

Up to 3 scan planes (generally at least para-axially and para-sagittally along the axis of the cannula) can be monitored with temperature mapping (T-maps) during the procedure. Additional planes increase the time between temperature updates.

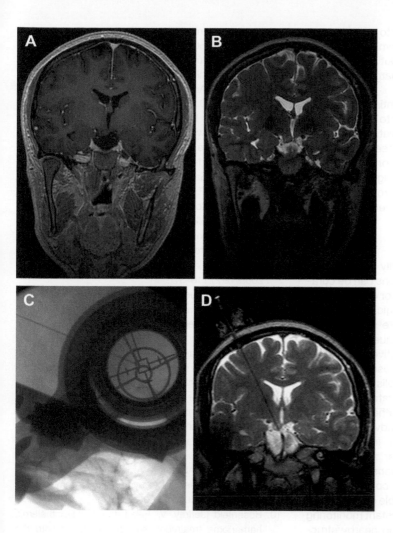

Fig. 7. MRI for case 2. (*A*) Coronal contrast-enhanced image showing right-sided HH. (*B*) Coronal T2-weighted image again depicting HH. (*C*) Intraoperative fluoroscopy showing cannula just above arc center in the Leksell frame. (*D*) Intraoperative T2-weighted MRI showing the cannula at target.

When the planes are established, the laser power source is attached to the optical fiber, and irrigation tubing is attached. Before proceeding, return flow of the irrigation should be confirmed.

Next, safety monitoring points are chosen. The temperature at up to 6 points can be monitored. Typically, 3 high points are chosen near the diffuser tip to ensure the temperature does not exceed 90°C, to protect the tip. Three points are chosen to automatically turn off the laser if temperature exceeds 45 to 50°C.

The laser is activated at 30% power (4.5 W) to verify the location of the diffuser tip. This can be translated in or out as needed. When this is confirmed, we proceed to ablation.

We typically create the first few overlapping ablations at 50–60% power. Each lesion is carried out until the pixels indicating the irreversible damage zone plateau, typically after 2 but no more than 3 minutes at a time. The cannula is then retracted 5 to 8 mm and overlapping ablations are serially performed as far back as needed to cover the tumor.

The immediate effects of the ablation are apparent on diffusion-weighted imaging, FLAIR (fluid-attenuated inversion recovery), T2, and gadolinium-enhanced T1 (eg, magnetization prepared rapid acquisition gradient echo; MPRAGE) imaging, the latter of which demonstrates the area of blood-brain barrier breakdown at the periphery of the lesion (see **Fig. 6**E, F).

When ablation is confirmed, the laser assembly and frame are removed. A single staple is used to close the skin incision.

Postablation Management

The patient typically is monitored for 1 night on a standard hospital unit. No intensive care unit monitoring is required in the absence of a complication. Steroids are administered for 1 to 2 weeks. A transient headache is a common complaint following the procedure; this may be related to inflammatory cytokines released by the lesion coming in contact with the dura (eg, tentorial edge), but also could be related to local mass effect. Discharge on the day after surgery is typical.

Antiepileptic medication is continued without change. We will taper medications to some degree (eg, decreasing dosage[s] or eliminating a medication) if the patient remains seizure free at 6 months, but will never discontinue medications completely until 2 years. Postoperative imaging beyond that acquired at the completion of the procedure is obtained only in the event of seizure recurrence.

SUMMARY AND DISCUSSION

HHs are rare lesions in a surgically fraught area. Resection or ablation of these lesions can be curative, not only for seizures but also for cognitive and behavioral deficits. Open surgical resection and endoscopic disconnection are successful in roughly half of cases, but have frequent complications. Radiosurgery is less effective, and takes many months before effects are observed.

Although there is only one published study of laser ablation for HHs,[20] the rate of seizure freedom appears higher than all other modalities, with potentially lower rates of adverse events. The 2 patients described earlier in this article were also seizure free after laser ablation, and neither had permanent complications.

The efficacy of laser ablation compared with other modalities has several possible explanations. First, MRI thermometry allows constant monitoring of thermal energy in the lesion and nearby structures. This allows constant assessment of the degree to which the lesion is damaged, and assessment of safety for surrounding structures. No other ablative modality currently provides this assurance. Second, the small surgical opening reduces the frequency of surgical complications, as compared with open and even endoscopic procedures, although there is always a chance of infection and hemorrhage with stereotactic procedures, no matter how small the entry point.

Overall, MRI-guided laser ablation appears to be a safe and effective means of treating HHs. Further surgical series are needed, but preliminary evidence is encouraging. As technology improves and more clinical data are acquired, laser ablation has the potential to supplant conventional treatments for this rare but morbid disease.

REFERENCES

1. Salvatore S, Pasquale S, Antonietta C, et al. The syndrome gelastic seizures–hypothalamic hamartoma: severe, potentially reversible encephalopathy. Epilepsia 2009;50(s5):62–5.
2. Boyko OB, Curnes JT, Oakes WJ, et al. Hamartomas of the tuber cinereum: CT, MR, and pathologic findings. AJNR Am J Neuroradiol 1991;12(2):309–14.
3. Delalande O, Fohlen M. Disconnecting surgical treatment of hypothalamic hamartoma in children and adults with refractory epilepsy and proposal of a new classification. Neurol Med Chir (Tokyo) 2003;43(2):61–8.
4. Berkovic Samuel F, Kuzniecky Ruben I, Andermann F. Human epileptogenesis and hypothalamic hamartomas: new lessons from an experiment of nature. Epilepsia 1997;38(1):1–3.
5. Kerrigan John F, Ng YT, Chung S, et al. The hypothalamic hamartoma: a model of subcortical epileptogenesis and encephalopathy. Semin Pediatr Neurol 2005;12(2):119–31.
6. Berkovic Samuel F, Alexis A, Ruben K, et al. Hypothalamic hamartoma and seizures: a treatable epileptic encephalopathy. Epilepsia 2003;44(7):969–73.
7. Striano S, Striano P, Sarappa C, et al. The clinical spectrum and natural history of gelastic epilepsy-hypothalamic hamartoma syndrome. Seizure 2005;14(4):232–9.
8. Fenoglio Kristina A, Jie W, Do Young K, et al. Hypothalamic hamartoma: basic mechanisms of intrinsic epileptogenesis. Semin Pediatr Neurol 2007;14(2):51–9.
9. Wait Scott D, Abla Adib A, Killory Brendan D, et al. Surgical approaches to hypothalamic hamartomas. Neurosurg Focus 2011;30(2):E2.
10. Rosenfeld Jeffrey V, Feiz-Erfan I. Hypothalamic hamartoma treatment: surgical resection with the transcallosal approach. Semin Pediatr Neurol 2007;14(2):88–98.
11. Rekate Harold L, Feiz-Erfan I, Ng YT, et al. Endoscopic surgery for hypothalamic hamartomas causing medically refractory gelastic epilepsy. Childs Nerv Syst 2006;22(8):874–80.
12. Ng YT, Rekate HL, Prenger EC, et al. Endoscopic resection of hypothalamic hamartomas for refractory symptomatic epilepsy. Neurology 2008;70(17):1543–8.
13. Kyu-Won S, Jong-Hee C, Yong-Gou P, et al. Treatment modality for intractable epilepsy in hypothalamic hamartomatous lesions. Neurosurgery 2008;62(4):847–56 [discussion: 856].
14. Shigeki K, Hiroatsu M, Hiroshi M, et al. Minimally invasive magnetic resonance imaging-guided stereotactic radiofrequency thermocoagulation for epileptogenic hypothalamic hamartomas. Neurosurgery 2009;65(3):438–49.
15. Kuzniecky Ruben I, Guthrie Barton L. Stereotactic surgical approach to hypothalamic hamartomas. Epileptic Disord 2003;5(4):275–80.

16. Jean R, Didier S, Manabu T, et al. Epilepsy related to hypothalamic hamartomas: surgical management with special reference to gamma knife surgery. Childs Nerv Syst 2006;22(8):881–95.

17. Akai T, Okamoto K, Iizuka H, et al. Treatments of hamartoma with neuroendoscopic surgery and stereotactic radiosurgery: a case report. Minim Invasive Neurosurg 2002;45(4):235–9.

18. Papayannis CE, Consalvo D, Seifer G, et al. Clinical spectrum and difficulties in management of hypothalamic hamartoma in a developing country. Acta Neurol Scand 2008;118(5):313–9.

19. Selch MT, Gorgulho A, Mattozo C, et al. Linear accelerator stereotactic radiosurgery for the treatment of gelastic seizures due to hypothalamic hamartoma. Minim Invasive Neurosurg 2005;48(5): 310–4.

20. Wilfong AA, Curry DJ. Hypothalamic hamartomas: Optimal approach to clinical evaluation and diagnosis. Epilepsia 2013;54(Suppl. 9):109–14.

Laser Ablation in Pediatric Epilepsy

Robert Buckley, MD[a], Samuel Estronza-Ojeda, MD[b], Jeffrey G. Ojemann, MD[a],*

KEYWORDS

- Pediatric epilepsy surgery • Laser ablation • Mesial temporal sclerosis • Hypothalamic hamartoma
- Neuropsychological outcome

KEY POINTS

- Laser ablation is a novel, minimally invasive technique for the surgical treatment of intractable epilepsy that involves MRI-guided thermal ablation of epileptogenic foci.
- Consider in patients with intractable epilepsy secondary to focal lesions, such as mesial temporal sclerosis, hypothalamic hamartomas, and possibly low-grade glioneuronal tumors.
- Early experience suggests less procedural morbidity, better neuropsychological outcomes, and similar short-term seizure freedom rates when compared with standard open surgical resection, but longer term study is needed.

INTRODUCTION

Pediatric epilepsy affects roughly 1 of every 100 children, of which as many of one-third have seizures that are incompletely controlled with medication alone. In children with medically intractable epilepsy who also have a radiographic and/or electrographic correlate for seizure origin, surgical resection is commonly considered.[1,2] In appropriately selected patients, long-term seizure control rates will be in the 50% to 70% range after removal of the epileptogenic focus. Conventional surgical treatment consists of an open surgical procedure (craniotomy) and resection of the offending tissue. Although extensive experience supports the efficacy and safety of this approach, the attendant risks of open surgery with regard to procedural morbidity, incomplete resection, and damage to adjacent brain tissue cannot be completely eliminated. This supports a role for minimally invasive alternatives when treating certain epileptogenic lesions, especially those adjacent to or involving deep or eloquent brain structures, such as the dominant temporal lobe and deep brain structures (eg, hypothalamic hamartoma [HH]).

Laser ablation is a novel, minimally invasive surgical technique[3] that is used in the treatment of focal, medically intractable pediatric epilepsy.[4] Previous attempts with stereotactic lesioning for the treatment of epilepsy were limited due to the variability in thermal energy delivery and inability to achieve real-time feedback on the area of ablated tissue.[5] Two systems, the Visualase[6,7] device (Medtronic, Minneapolis, MN) and the Monteris device (Plymouth, MN),[8] have recently been used for ablation of seizure foci. Generally, both systems consist of a laser catheter probe that is placed by the neurosurgeon into a previously identified epileptogenic focus via a small twist-drill cranial access site. The surgeon can then use real-time MRI thermal imaging to visualize treatment and tailor the ablation to encompass the entirety of the lesion while avoiding surrounding critical brain structures.

Early use of this approach in children with epilepsy[4] shows its feasibility. It is particularly attractive for lesions such as HHs, in which the approach to the lesion can carry much of the morbidity. Deep heterotopia also may be targeted.[9] Additionally, following the experience in adults, ablation of the dominant temporal hippocampus

[a] Department of Neurological Surgery, Seattle Children's Hospital, University of Washington, 4800 Sand Point Way NE, Seattle, WA 98145-5005, USA; [b] Division of Neurosurgery, Seattle Children's Hospital, University of Puerto Rico, San Juan, PR, USA
* Corresponding author.
E-mail address: jojemann@u.washington.edu

Neurosurg Clin N Am 27 (2016) 69–78
http://dx.doi.org/10.1016/j.nec.2015.08.006

may provide improved neuropsychological outcomes compared with even selective resections.[10]

PATIENT EVALUATION

Pediatric patients with focal, medically intractable epilepsy are considered for possible surgical treatment to include laser ablation. Children whose seizures are inadequately controlled on 2 or more antiepileptic medications meet criteria for intractable epilepsy and warrant additional workup for possible surgical treatment.

Initial evaluation of patients with new-onset epilepsy consists of assessment by a pediatric epileptologist with scalp electroencephalogram (EEG) and pharmacologic therapy, as deemed appropriate. High-resolution MRI is obtained to identify any potential underlying structural abnormalities, such as hippocampal sclerosis, HHs, gray matter heterotopia, cortical dysplasia, or masses that may represent the origin for the child's seizures. All patients considered for surgery undergo long-term video EEG monitoring to provide additional information regarding seizure localization and semiology and attempt to correlate seizure origin with any relevant radiographic findings. Neuropsychological testing is performed to assist in identification of dysfunction that is relevant for localization, and preoperative consultations, especially for surgery in proximity to key structures involved in cognition, language, and memory, such as the dominant mesial temporal lobe. PET is frequently used and additional modalities are used as needed. Functional MRI is commonly used to assist in localization of function and assessment of reorganization from presumed seizure foci.[11]

After evaluation in a multidisciplinary epilepsy conference, children with radiographic and electrographic correlation with a candidate epileptogenic focus amenable to surgery are referred for neurosurgical evaluation. Invasive monitoring may be needed to define the seizure-onset zone if the remainder of the evaluation is incongruent. In our pediatric population, the most common indications for laser ablation are mesial temporal sclerosis, HHs, and other focal lesions to include low-grade glioneuronal tumors, such as ganglioglioma and dysembryoplastic neuroepithelial tumor (DNET). Specific considerations regarding patient selection and evaluation are described for each of these in the following sections.

Mesial Temporal Sclerosis

Mesial temporal sclerosis (MTS) is of one of the most commonly encountered focal epilepsy pathologies. MTS may have a higher incidence of associated pathology (dual pathology) in the pediatric population.[12] Radiographic findings consist of hippocampal signal change, loss of internal architecture, and/or volume loss on the affected side. Histopathologically confirmed MTS may have subtle imaging findings.[13]

In these children, both open temporal lobectomy and laser ablation of the mesial temporal structures offer a reasonable approach to treatment, and they are used concurrently in our practice. Based on the adult experience of less cognitive decrement with laser ablation,[10] we will typically offer laser ablation to those with suspected isolated dominant temporal lobe MTS foci. Semiology, EEG, or imaging features that suggest dual pathology would require either a larger resection or a limited treatment only after the use of invasive monitoring.

In adult patients with dominant mesial temporal lobe epilepsy, the experience at our and other institutions suggests that laser ablation offers improved neuropsychological outcomes when compared with standard open temporal lobectomy. A recent series[10] of adult patients undergoing laser ablation for mesial temporal lobe epilepsy had significant preservation of famous face and common noun naming when compared with similar patients undergoing open temporal lobectomy.

In children, in whom there is concern for lateral temporal or extratemporal contribution to seizures on electrographic and/or radiographic evaluation, targeted laser ablation of the mesial temporal structures would be less effective in achieving acceptable seizure control. With nondominant temporal lobe involvement, the use of laser ablation would be balanced by the relatively good cognitive outcome with anterior temporal lobectomy and the concern of lower seizure control with a more limited treatment.

Laser ablation additionally offers patients and their families a less invasive approach to surgical management of intractable mesial temporal epilepsy. In patients in whom either laser ablation or standard open resection offers near equivalence in treatment benefits and risks, the preference of the child and his or her parents is a valid selection criterion. In our experience, the potential of a less-invasive treatment modality has allowed us to treat patients who would otherwise refuse open surgery.

Hypothalamic Hamartomas

HHs represent a rare congenital malformation involving the hypothalamus that present with a characteristic epilepsy syndrome. Seizures are classically gelastic type, which are characterized by spells of laughing and altered mental status. Gelastic seizures are notoriously medication-resistant and children with HHs can progress to epileptic encephalopathy with attendant impairments in behavior and cognition. Treatment of HHs with associated intractable epilepsy has been with open and endoscopic surgical resection.[14] Based on their deep location and intimate association with the hypothalamus and other associated critical brain structures, surgery for these lesions carries not insignificant risks, to include endocrine dysfunction, weight gain, memory impairment, and even coma.

In children with HHs, we have moved to regarding laser ablation as first-line therapy. Laser ablation offers the benefit of minimal brain manipulation when compared with open and endoscopic surgical approaches. It additionally has the benefit of allowing real-time assessment of the area of thermal treatment; this provides the surgeon increased control, which is key when working adjacent to deep brain structures.

Low-Grade Glioneuronal Tumors

Low-grade glial neoplasms, such as ganglioglioma and DNET, represent an additional source of focal epilepsy in children. The most common presentation is seizures, which are commonly resistant to antiepileptic medication. Surgical management of these lesions is variable; children with intractable epilepsy usually undergo surgical management, which is effective in approximately 70% or more in providing seizure control.

Laser ablation is an alternative to standard open resection of these lesions. Recent literature supports the effectiveness of laser ablation in treating primary glial neoplasms[15,16] and brain metastases[17] in the adult population. We consider the use of laser ablation in children with these low-grade glial tumors and resultant intractable epilepsy in certain cases. The stereotactic frame used in placement of the laser catheter also can be used to obtain core tissue biopsies for pathology before thermal ablation. Also, the laser system can be used for treatment of multifocal lesions or in combination with a standard laser amygdalohippocampectomy in children with combined pathology.

LASER ABLATION
Surgical Technique

Anesthesia
A standard endotracheal intubation is performed with total intravenous anesthesia infusion of propofol and fentanyl with fine adjustment of sevoflurane, to allow for a motionless patient. An important

aspect throughout the procedure is adequate analgesia and body temperature management, especially during patient transport. Important adjunct parts of anesthesia include the administration of preoperative antibiotics within 1 hour of incision. Other aspects of preoperative preparation include adequate placement of peripheral intravenous lines and insertion of urinary catheter for proper fluid management. Steroids are administered before performing the ablation to decrease treatment-associated edema, with dosing of dexamethasone at approximately 0.2 mg/kg up to 10 mg intravenously as a single dose, with a wide range of specific dosing possible based on practice preference. Active warming is used when the patient is not in transport or in the scanner.

Procedure
After endotracheal anesthesia is initiated, the Cosman-Roberts-Wells (CRW) frame is placed with the use of local anesthesia on pin sites (**Fig. 1**). The patient is then transported to the radiology department for registration/planning study. For patients undergoing ablation on tumors or other similar lesions, a half-dose contrast-enhancing brain MRI is performed. Only half-dose contrast is administered on this initial brain MRI to be able to give contrast again on the posttreatment study. On patients with hamartomas or MTS, computed tomography (CT) of the head without contrast is performed and subsequently merged with a recent brain MRI. After the appropriated study has been performed, the patient is returned to the operating room (OR).

Back in the OR, the planning study is uploaded to the Medtronic Stealth Station (Framelink) or equivalent planning software. After successful

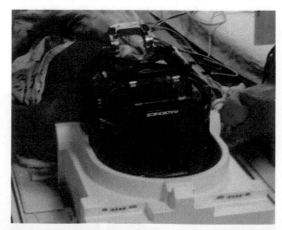

Fig. 1. The stereotactic frame is placed and the child is taken, under anesthesia, to either the MRI or CT scan for a localizing study.

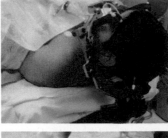
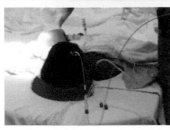
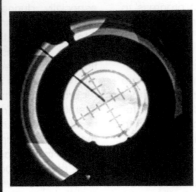

Fig. 2. The patient, in the frame, is secured to the table (*upper left panel*). The arc is placed on the frame and the laser passed through a 3.2-mm drill hole. Fluoroscopic guidance demonstrates the correct targeting of the laser stylet to the frame target (*right frame*). The frame is carefully removed and the laser sits in the skull bolt (*lower left frame*).

registration, we select the target, trajectory, and entry point best suited to the case, avoiding when possible the ventricular system and traversing vessels. The resulting CRW coordinates are entered in the CRW Precision Arc (Integra Health, Inc., Plainsboro, NJ, USA) and accuracy confirmed with the CRW Phantom base. After the patient is appropriately positioned on the Mayfield (Integra LifeSciences, Plainsboro, NJ, USA) adaptor, prepped and draped, the Precision Arc is placed on the frame. Then the C-Arm is brought in, and aligned with the arc rings for later X-ray confirmation of target.

The CRW trajectory determines the entry point at which the incision is made and the skull is drilled with a 3.2-mm drill bit. After the skull is appropriately drilled and dura opened, the Precision Arc is used to introduce the stylet through the selected entry point and trajectory, with subsequent C-Arm confirmation of arrival at the target. Then the stylet is removed and a PMT (Chanhassen, MN, USA) bolt is placed in the skull for later catheter and laser fixation. Following adequate bolt placement,

under fluoroscopic guidance, the laser sheath is placed to target location. After the catheter and laser are fixed with the bolt, the Precision Arc is removed from the frame, the patient taken out of the Mayfield adapter, and the frame removed from the patient (**Fig. 2**).

Following the removal of the stereotactic equipment, the patient is transported to the 3T MRI suite for treatment. On arrival, the patient is placed in the MRI, and the catheter and laser connected to the Visualase system. Before treatment is started, sagittal and axial views of the laser are performed on a T1 sequence MRI for location confirmation (**Fig. 3**). When placing more than one catheter, one should always be aware of the proximity of the distal tips to avoid possible malfunction and unwanted complications (**Fig. 4**). After confirmation of laser location, the MRI is coupled with the Visualase system, which provides continuous MR thermography imaging for real-time thermal monitoring. Following the transfer of images to the Visualase system, we proceed to select our target area and safety margins appropriate to the case.

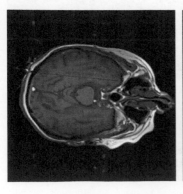
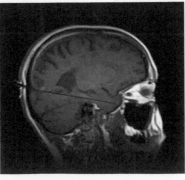

Fig. 3. The catheter is monitored in orthogonal planes. The source image is on the left and the (T1-weighted) anatomic image is used for reference on the right.

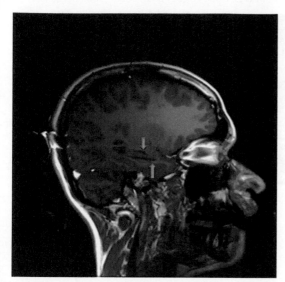

Fig. 4. Two catheters are used (*arrows*). Care is taken to minimize overlap between the two, and cooling with the saline that runs around the catheter is mandatory to prevent damage to the adjacent catheter during treatment.

The selected target area will reach the predetermined treatment temperature for the pathology at hand, which should be between 50°C and 90°C for adequate tissue coagulation. On the other hand, if the temperature on the selected safety margins reaches the critical level of approximately 45°C, the laser will shut off, avoiding damage to those areas, because if temperature is kept below the critical level, thermal damage will not occur, regardless of exposure time. These selected markers allow for precise target coagulation, avoiding damage to important surrounding brain tissue.

Laser treatment is started with a low-power trial (~30%) to ensure adequate laser function and location. After a successful trial, we proceed with the ablation at the power and temperature adequate for the case. For example, we approach narrow-diameter target lesions with quick high-power ablations, and wide-diameter target lesions with slow low-power ablations. For target lesions not fully covered by the length of the laser tip, we perform multiple contiguous ablations by retracting the laser approximately 1 mm after each attempt until complete ablation of the target lesion is seen in the combined damage model. During the entire procedure, we are constantly monitoring the live temperature maps and real-time damage model, and making the necessary adjustments to precisely ablate the target lesion and minimize the risk of potential damage to the healthy brain tissue (**Fig. 5**).

Immediately after completion of the laser treatment, a contrast-enhancing brain MRI is performed emphasizing postcontrast T1, fluid-attenuated inversion recovery (FLAIR), and diffusion tensor imaging for adequate posttreatment evaluation and confirmation of target lesion ablation (**Fig. 6**). Following posttreatment study, the

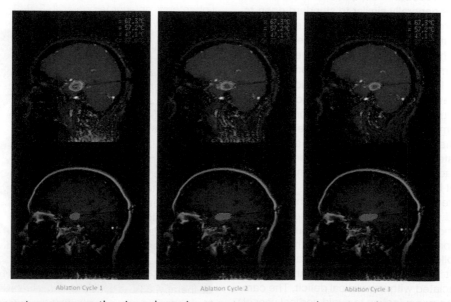

Fig. 5. Temperature maps use the phase dependence on temperature to determine relative heating. A damage estimate map is superimposed on the earlier anatomic study. Tissue that has received heating such that permanent damage is expected is indicated by orange.

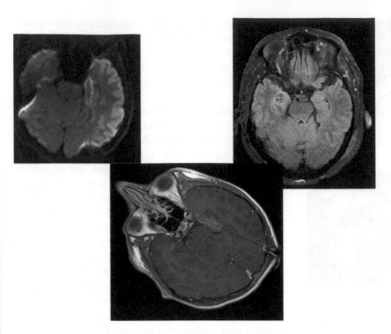

Fig. 6. Examples from different pediatric patients with hippocampal ablation showing restricted diffusion in the left hippocampus (*upper left panel*), FLAIR signal change in the right hippocampus (*upper right panel*), and enhancement in the ablation region (*lower panel*).

patient is transported to the recovery room for sterile removal of the laser, catheter, and PMT bolt, with subsequent wound closure. If no complications occur, the patient is discharged in 24 hours to standard outpatient follow-up and a follow-up MRI study performed generally within 6 to 12 weeks.

COMPLICATIONS

In theory, procedural complications from laser ablation are generally similar to standard open resective surgery, with a few notable exceptions. When counseling children and their families regarding the risks of laser ablation, we note risks of symptomatic hemorrhage, infection, cerebrospinal fluid leak (especially if the ventricle is transversed), device complications, neurologic deficit, failure to cure, stroke, and death. In practice, the risk of damage to nearby vessels seems to be less, as heat does not appear to accumulate around cisterns (**Fig. 7**) and visual fibers are minimally impacted by this approach compared with a temporal lobe resection.

We have not seen symptomatic hemorrhage associated with the passing of the laser catheter, although most patients have minimal susceptibility artifact representing hemorrhage in the catheter tract on follow-up MRI scans; this is an unavoidable result of the procedure itself, and has not been associated with any clinical deficit. The careful use of neuronavigation to avoid cortical vessels and deep vascular structures is important in helping to minimize this risk of serious hemorrhage.

Postoperative infections, either intracranial or wound, have not been seen in our series of pediatric patients receiving laser ablation. Cerebrospinal fluid leak also remains a theoretic risk in children undergoing laser ablation. Interestingly, we have used laser ablation over open resection in a number of patients with baseline ventriculomegaly and concern for arrested hydrocephalus (**Fig. 8**); this

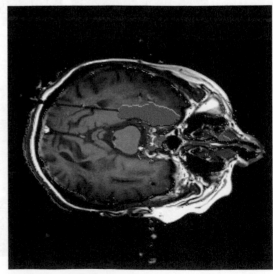

Fig. 7. Temperature map is highly conformal, avoiding heating of the ventricle or of the cistern and sulci medially.

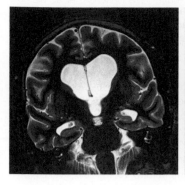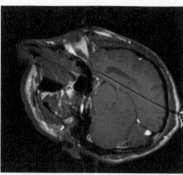

Fig. 8. Arrested hydrocephalus and hippocampal sclerosis. Laser ablation avoids exposing the ventricle, as would be needed in a temporal lobectomy, no matter how selective.

allows us to avoid entering the ventricular system and the introduction of postsurgical blood products that can result in delayed hydrocephalus.

Unsurprisingly, as we develop our initial experience with laser ablation, we have seen a number of procedural complications. Most common of these are failure of the bolt system, leading to retained fragments; we have had 2 adult patients require return to the OR for removal of such. One pediatric patient undergoing ablation of an HH had deflection of the laser catheter when attempting to enter the lesion; this was noted on initial localization MR imaging (**Fig. 9**). The patient was brought back to the OR and the catheter was replaced in the proper location and ablation proceeded uneventfully.

Transient or permanent neurologic deficit is a significant potential complication to any surgical treatment of epilepsy, including laser ablation. In our pediatric patients we have not seen significant postoperative neurologic deficit after ablation of

the mesial temporal structures or cortical tumors. In those children undergoing ablation of HHs, transient hemiparesis was seen in 2 patients; one of these had stuttering on delayed postoperative follow-up of unclear etiology. These were both thought to be due to proximity of the treatment zone to the internal capsule. An additional patient with HH had transient blurred vision that responded to a several-day course of steroids. No specific abnormalities on MRI posttreatment were identIfled; our belief is that this may be secondary to local thermal effects and/or edema with a mild ventriculitis.

We have not experienced procedural mortality or other devastating complications in our patients undergoing laser ablation. Although we remain in

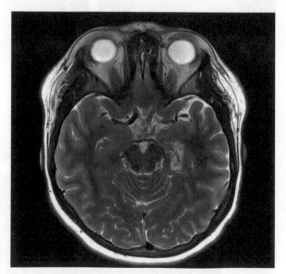

Fig. 10. Axial T2-weighted MRI 6 months postablation. The seizures returned and, on invasive monitoring, the focus came from the anterior aspect of the medial temporal lobe, just at the margin of the previous ablation, which was insufficient in anterior extent.

Fig. 9. Misplacement of the catheter, intended to target the HH. The catheter was repositioned and the hamartoma ablated.

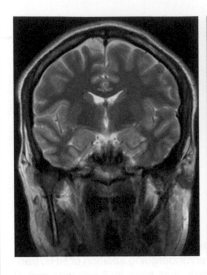

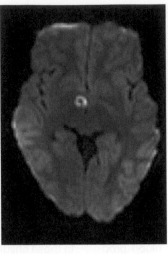

Fig. 11. HH and postablation images demonstrating ablation of the lesion.

the early stages of our experience with the procedure, it is clear that complications associated with laser ablation are at least comparable and potentially more favorable when compared with open resective surgery.

OUTCOMES

Although limited by the lack of long-term follow-up, outcomes in pediatric patients undergoing laser ablation for intractable epilepsy are generally good, with seizure control rates near-equivalent to

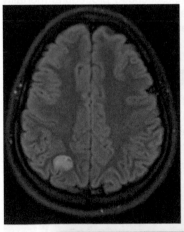

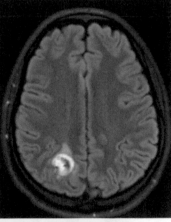

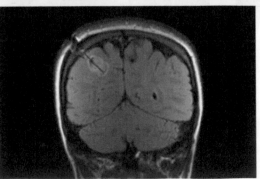

Fig. 12. A right parietal lesion (*left*) biopsied at the same setting as placement of the laser catheter. The pathology was DNET and the ablation (*bottom*) and postablation (*right*) panels demonstrate the ablation effect. Patient is seizure free and deficit free at 6 months out.

those for corresponding open resective procedures.

In children undergoing surgical therapy for treatment of medically intractable mesial temporal lobe epilepsy, extensive literature supports a seizure control rate of 60% to 80% depending on patient characteristics.[1] In our experience, all patients had at least some benefit in terms of seizure reduction (Engel class 3) with approximately 50% of patients seizure free (Engel class 1) at time of last follow-up. Whether this will represent long-term outcomes and the influence of patient characteristics will be better understood with increasing volumes at our institution and others.

Neuropsychological outcomes, such as naming and verbal and working memory, appear significantly better in our pediatric patients undergoing laser ablation when compared with open temporal lobectomy, although loss of verbal memory function can be seen. Despite the increased risk of failure to control seizures after laser ablation, it is our feeling that the neuropsychological benefits support making it the first-line therapy for dominant mesial temporal lobe epilepsy. Laser ablation additionally preserves the ability to perform a standard anterior temporal lobectomy if seizures persist.

In one instructive case, seizures recurred after mesial temporal ablation (**Fig. 10**). Invasive monitoring localized the seizures to the anterior boundaries of the resection. The family did not wish repeat ablation and surgical resection was performed. The laser cavity was firm and gliotic, but with no surrounding distortion of the anatomy, allowing for routine resection of remaining mesial structures and seizure freedom following surgery.

Seizure control rates in our patients undergoing laser ablation of HHs (**Fig. 11**) and focal cortical lesions (**Fig. 12**) are similar to that for open resection, with Engel class 1 results in approximately 75% and 65%, respectively, again with short-term follow-up only.

Even if outcomes undergoing laser ablation in our institutional experience and the published literature are slightly decreased with regard to improved neuropsychological outcomes, this represents a favorable tradeoff for initial surgical therapy in our pediatric patients. Long-term outcome data are still lacking, and will be critical in guiding the use of laser ablation in the coming years.

REFERENCES

1. Ojemann J. Temporal lobe epilepsy. In: Albright AL, Pollack IF, Adelson PD, editors. Principles and practice of pediatric neurosurgery. New York: Thieme; 2014.

2. Russ SA, Larson K, Halfon N. A national profile of childhood epilepsy and seizure disorder. Pediatrics 2012;129(2):256–64.

3. McNichols RJ, Gowda A, Kangasniemi M, et al. MR thermometry-based feedback control of laser interstitial thermal therapy at 980 nm. Lasers Surg Med 2004;34(1):48–55.

4. Curry DJ, Gowda A, McNichols RJ, et al. MR-guided stereotactic laser ablation of epileptogenic foci in children. Epilepsy Behav 2012;24(4):408–14.

5. Quigg M, Harden C. Minimally invasive techniques for epilepsy surgery: stereotactic radiosurgery and other technologies. J Neurosurg 2014;121(Suppl): 232–40.

6. Tovar-Spinoza Z, Carter D, Ferrone D, et al. The use of MRI-guided laser-induced thermal ablation for epilepsy. Childs Nerv Syst 2013;29(11):2089–94.

7. Willie JT, Laxpati NG, Drane DL, et al. Real-time magnetic resonance-guided stereotactic laser amygdalohippocampotomy for mesial temporal lobe epilepsy. Neurosurgery 2014;74(6):569–84.

8. Hawasli AH, Bandt SK, Hogan RE, et al. Laser ablation as treatment strategy for medically refractory dominant insular epilepsy: therapeutic and functional considerations. Stereotact Funct Neurosurg 2014;92(6):397–404.

9. Esquenazi Y, Kalamangalam GP, Slater JD, et al. Stereotactic laser ablation of epileptogenic periventricular nodular heterotopia. Epilepsy Res 2014; 108(3):547–54.

10. Drane DL, Loring DW, Voets NL, et al. Better object recognition and naming outcome with MRI-guided stereotactic laser amygdalohippocampotomy for temporal lobe epilepsy. Epilepsia 2015;56(1): 101–13.

11. Shurtleff H, Warner M, Poliakov A, et al. Functional magnetic resonance imaging for presurgical evaluation of very young pediatric patients with epilepsy. J Neurosurg Pediatr 2010;5(5):500–6.

12. Mohamed A, Wyllie E, Ruggieri P, et al. Temporal lobe epilepsy due to hippocampal sclerosis in pediatric candidates for epilepsy surgery. Neurology 2001;56(12):1643–9.

13. Kasasbeh A, Hwang EC, Steger-May K, et al. Association of magnetic resonance imaging identification of mesial temporal sclerosis with pathological diagnosis and surgical outcomes in children following epilepsy surgery. J Neurosurg Pediatr 2012;9(5): 552–61.

14. Wait SD, Abla AA, Killory BD, et al. Surgical approaches to hypothalamic hamartomas. Neurosurg Focus 2011;30(2):E2.

15. Mohammadi AM, Hawasli AH, Rodriguez A, et al. The role of laser interstitial thermal therapy in enhancing progression-free survival of difficult-to-access high-grade gliomas: a multicenter study. Cancer Med 2014;3(4):971–9.

16. Sloan AE, Ahluwalia MS, Valerio-Pascua J, et al. Results of the NeuroBlate System first-in-humans Phase I clinical trial for recurrent glioblastoma: clinical article. J Neurosurg 2013; 118(6):1202–19.

17. Carpentier A, McNichols RJ, Stafford RJ, et al. Laser thermal therapy: real-time MRI-guided and computer-controlled procedures for metastatic brain tumors. Lasers Surg Med 2011;43(10): 943–50.

Radiosurgery for Medial Temporal Lobe Epilepsy Resulting from Mesial Temporal Sclerosis

Thomas Gianaris, MD, Thomas Witt, MD, Nicholas M. Barbaro, MD*

KEYWORDS

- Mesial temporal sclerosis • Medial temporal lobe epilepsy • Radiosurgery • Epilepsy

KEY POINTS

- Radiosurgery for mesial temporal sclerosis (MTS)–associated medial temporal lobe epilepsy (MTLE) is an attractive option because it is relatively noninvasive, with lower morbidity than major surgery.
- Conventional open temporal lobectomy surgery may also be pursued if initial radiosurgical treatment is ineffective and after sufficient time has been permitted for the delayed radiosurgical antiepileptic effect after 3 years.
- The main known disadvantage of radiosurgery at present is the delayed response for seizure control, during which time patients continue to suffer from the sequelae of seizures.
- Future research into radiosurgery modality will ideally make individualized patient treatment more feasible and attainable, allowing the neurosurgical community to more effectively manage and treat medial temporal lobe epilepsy.

INTRODUCTION

Radiosurgery is the precise application of focused radiation to targeted brain with the aid of stereotactic guidance.[1–27] Radiosurgery is particularly well suited for treatment of MTS leading to medial temporal lobe epilepsy because MTS typically exhibits radiographic changes on MRI, allowing this focused radiation to be directed to a specific, small region of pathology, sparing the rest of the brain from harmful radiation.[24] Regis and colleagues[28] were able to demonstrate the safety of focused radiosurgery for medial temporal lobe epilepsy while still delivering doses effective enough to reduce seizure frequency, whereas a prospective multicenter European study using the Gamma Knife proprietary radiosurgery tools found similar efficacy rates for seizure reduction with a dose of 29 Gy, comparing radiosurgery to the gold standard of conventional microsurgery for epilepsy after 2 years with similar morbidity and mortality.

A similar multicenter trial studying a direct comparison of radiosurgery to resection for MTLE has shown in pilot studies that a dose of 24 Gy to the medial temporal lobe was able to eliminate seizures in 85% of patients at 2 years of follow-up as well.[29] In this pilot study, patients were treated with 2 different radiation doses (20 Gy or 24 Gy) and there was significant seizure remission in both groups at 12 months (58.8% and 76.9%, respectively), with no dose-based or seizure remission–based changes in headaches, visual field defects, and the use of steroids. Although these studies thus far only have time points at 1

Department of Neurological Surgery, Indiana University School of Medicine, 355 W. 16th St., Suite 5100, Indianapolis, IN 46202, USA
* Corresponding author.
E-mail address: Nbarbaro@iupui.edu

Neurosurg Clin N Am 27 (2016) 79–82
http://dx.doi.org/10.1016/j.nec.2015.08.011
1042-3680/16/$ – see front matter © 2016 Elsevier Inc. All rights reserved.

and 2 years, recent research in France looking at outcomes of 5 and 8 years has demonstrated continued seizure reduction remission after radiosurgery, although at a lower rate, finding 47% remission at 5 years and 60% at 8 years.[30,31] In addition, there may be benefits with respect to memory and language preservation.

RISKS OF TREATMENT

Although these studies have shown that radiosurgery is effective with minimal morbidity and mortality at time points of greater than 1 year, radiosurgery, unlike open resection, has a lag time after treatment before patients begin to see the effects of therapy and, in the near term, patients are still exposed to the risks of continued seizures as well as the risks of radiation. Typically, patients treated with radiosurgery can achieve seizure reduction at 9 to 12 months and possible complete cessation of seizures between 18 and 24 months after radiosurgery treatment.[28] In addition, a transient increase in partial seizures (auras) can be noted at approximately the same time that complex seizures decrease with radiosurgery, and many of them require a transient period of steroid administration for the radiation-induced edema.[28] Srikijvilaikul and colleagues[32] found 2 deaths during this latency period in a small case series of 5 patients treated with 20 Gy before seizure remission, likely complications of ongoing seizures. Quigg and colleagues[33] found that language (Boston Naming Test), verbal memory (California Verbal Learning Test and Logical Memory Subtest of the Wechsler Memory Scale—Revised), cognitive efficiency and mental flexibility (Trail Making Test), and mood (Beck Depression Inventory) did not differ from baseline after radiosurgery, demonstrating long-term neurocognitive safety using established scoring scales, despite the increased potential for necrosis.

Radiosurgery for MTLE is not without risks and long-term effects; radiation necrosis has been demonstrated by several studies and case reports. Hensley-Judge and colleagues[34] found postoperative visual field deficits in 15 of 24 (62.5%) patients, all homonymous superior quadrantanopias, proportions similar to historical comparisons from open surgery for MTLE. Another case series demonstrated that 2 of 7 patients, status postradiosurgery for MTS presenting with symptomatic radiation necrosis, required resection after 5 and 10 years.[35] Additionally, there is some concern in the long term for radiosurgery-associated radiation-induced malignancies, although these reported cases are rare, and none has been reported after therapy for MTS.[36–39] Although it was initially studied as a primary modality for MTS treatment, radiosurgery is also being investigated as a treatment of refractory epilepsy after temporal lobe resection. Yen and colleagues[40] found significant seizure reduction in a case series of 4 patients who underwent radiosurgery after temporal lobe resection. There was reduction of seizure frequency at 6 months after radiosurgery for refractory epilepsy after temporal lobe resection as well as improved neuropsychological profiles, including memory function and quality of life, lasting up to the 2-year follow-up examination.

MECHANISM OF ACTION AND HISTOPATHOLOGY

Conversely, open resective surgery after radiosurgery has, as a side benefit, provided an opportunity to understand the mechanism of action of radiosurgery on a histopathologic level. In 2 separate studies, Kawai and colleagues[41] and Srikijvilaikul and colleagues[32] found histologic changes, including necrotic foci with vessel wall thickening and fibrinoid and hyaline degeneration, in a patient treated with 18 Gy, as well as perivascular sclerosis and macrophage infiltration on resection and evaluation of a patient treated with 20 Gy. Cmelak and colleagues[42] reported no radiation-induced histopathologic changes in tissues treated with 15 Gy of radiosurgery, suggesting that some histologic damage may be needed for effective seizure control.[43–45] Chang and colleagues[46] found vasogenic edema appeared approximately 9 to 12 months after radiosurgery on serial MRI scans and correlated with the onset of seizure remission, further corroborating this hypothesis. Barbaro and colleagues[29] suggested that the mechanisms may be some combination of neuromodulation and true neuronal destruction, with some animal studies demonstrating improvement in seizures without evidence of necrosis, whereas other investigators have shown direct structural, destructive lesions in the tissue zone to correlate better with outcome, perhaps because of some contribution from ischemic factors.[46,47] The concrete mechanism of radiosurgery, destructive or otherwise, warrants further study.

SUMMARY

In summary, radiosurgery for MTS-associated MTLE is an attractive option because it is relatively noninvasive, with lower morbidity than major surgery. Conventional open temporal lobectomy surgery may also be pursued if the initial radiosurgical treatment is ineffective and after sufficient time has been permitted for the delayed radiosurgical antiepileptic effect after 3 years.[28] Its main known disadvantage at present is the delayed response for seizure control, during which time patients continue to suffer from the sequelae of seizures. Future research into this treatment modality will ideally make individualized patient treatment more feasible and attainable, allowing the neurosurgical community to more effectively manage and treat medial temporal lobe epilepsy.

REFERENCES

1. Engel J Jr. Surgery for seizures. N Engl J Med 1996; 334:647–52.
2. Wiebe S, Blume WT, Girvin JP, et al, Effectiveness, Efficiency of Surgery for Temporal Lobe Epilepsy Study Group. A randomized, controlled trial of surgery for temporal-lobe epilepsy. N Engl J Med 2001;345:311–8.
3. Bien CG, Kurthen M, Baron K, et al. Long-term seizure outcome and antiepileptic drug treatment in surgically treated temporal lobe epilepsy patients: a controlled study. Epilepsia 2001;42:1416–21.
4. Cascino GD. Clinical correlations with hippocampal atrophy. Magn Reson Imaging 1995;13:1133–6.
5. Cascino GD. Structural neuroimaging in partial epilepsy. Magnetic resonance imaging. Neurosurg Clin N Am 1995;6:455–64.
6. Engel J Jr. Update on surgical treatment of the epilepsies. Summary of the Second International Palm Desert Conference on the Surgical Treatment of the Epilepsies (1992). Neurology 1993;43:1612–7.
7. Garcia PA, Laxer KD, Barbaro NM, et al. Prognostic value of qualitative magnetic resonance imaging hippocampal abnormalities in patients undergoing temporal lobectomy for medically refractory seizures. Epilepsia 1994;35:520–4.
8. Spencer SS. Long-term outcome after epilepsy surgery. Epilepsia 1996;37:807–13.
9. Spencer SS, Berg AT, Vickrey BG, et al. Predicting long-term seizure outcome after resective epilepsy surgery: the multicenter study. Neurology 2005;65: 912–8.
10. Spencer SS, Berg AT, Vickrey BG, et al. Initial outcomes in the Multicenter Study of Epilepsy Surgery. Neurology 2003;61:1680–5.
11. Behrens E, Schramm J, Zentner J, et al. Surgical and neurological complications in a series of 708 epilepsy surgery procedures. Neurosurgery 1997; 41:1–9 [discussion: 9–10].
12. Rydenhag B, Silander HC. Complications of epilepsy surgery after 654 procedures in Sweden, September 1990-1995: a multicenter study based on the Swedish National Epilepsy Surgery Register. Neurosurgery 2001;49:51–6 [discussion: 56–7].
13. Siegel AM, Cascino GD, Meyer FB, et al. Surgical outcome and predictive factors in adult patients with intractable epilepsy and focal cortical dysplasia. Acta Neurol Scand 2006;113:65–71.
14. Sperling MR, Feldman H, Kinman J, et al. Seizure control and mortality in epilepsy. Ann Neurol 1999; 46:45–50.
15. Guldvog B, Loyning Y, Hauglie-Hanssen E, et al. Surgical versus medical treatment for epilepsy. II. Outcome related to social areas. Epilepsia 1991; 32:477–86.
16. Guldvog B, Loyning Y, Hauglie-Hanssen E, et al. Surgical versus medical treatment for epilepsy. I. Outcome related to survival, seizures, and neurologic deficit. Epilepsia 1991;32:375–88.
17. Barcia Salorio JL, Roldan P, Hernandez G, et al. Radiosurgical treatment of epilepsy. Appl Neurophysiol 1985;48:400–3.
18. Barcia-Salorio JL, Vanaclocha V, Cerda M, et al. Response of experimental epileptic focus to focal ionizing radiation. Appl Neurophysiol 1987;50:359–64.
19. Kitchen N. Experimental and clinical studies on the putative therapeutic efficacy of cerebral irradiation (radiotherapy) in epilepsy. Epilepsy Res 1995;20: 1–10.
20. Sun B, DeSalles AA, Medin PM, et al. Reduction of hippocampal-kindled seizure activity in rats by stereotactic radiosurgery. Exp Neurol 1998;154:691–5.
21. Herynek V, Burian M, Jirak D, et al. Metabolite and diffusion changes in the rat brain after Leksell Gamma Knife irradiation. Magn Reson Med 2004; 52:397–402.
22. Jirak D, Namestkova K, Herynek V, et al. Lesion evolution after gamma knife irradiation observed by magnetic resonance imaging. Int J Radiat Biol 2007;83:237–44.
23. Mori Y, Kondziolka D, Balzer J, et al. Effects of stereotactic radiosurgery on an animal model of hippocampal epilepsy. Neurosurgery 2000;46:157–65 [discussion: 165–8].
24. Dillon WP, Barbaro N. Noninvasive surgery for epilepsy: the era of image guidance. AJNR Am J Neuroradiol 1999;20:185.
25. Kondziolka D, Lunsford LD, Witt TC, et al. The future of radiosurgery: radiobiology, technology, and applications. Surg Neurol 2000;54:406–14.
26. Nguyen DK, Spencer SS. Recent advances in the treatment of epilepsy. Arch Neurol 2003;60:929–35.
27. Cohen-Gadol AA, Wilhelmi BG, Collignon F, et al. Long-term outcome of epilepsy surgery among 399 patients with nonlesional seizure foci including mesial temporal lobe sclerosis. J Neurosurg 2006; 104:513–24.
28. Regis J, Rey M, Bartolomei F, et al. Gamma knife surgery in mesial temporal lobe epilepsy: a prospective multicenter study. Epilepsia 2004;45:504–15.
29. Barbaro NM, Quigg M, Broshek DK, et al. A multicenter, prospective pilot study of gamma knife radiosurgery for mesial temporal lobe epilepsy:

seizure response, adverse events, and verbal memory. Ann Neurol 2009;65:167–75.

30. Bartolomei F, Hayashi M, Tamura M, et al. Long-term efficacy of gamma knife radiosurgery in mesial temporal lobe epilepsy. Neurology 2008;70:1658–63.

31. Rheims S, Fischer C, Ryvlin P, et al. Long-term outcome of gamma-knife surgery in temporal lobe epilepsy. Epilepsy Res 2008;80:23–9.

32. Srikijvilaikul T, Najm I, Foldvary-Schaefer N, et al. Failure of gamma knife radiosurgery for mesial temporal lobe epilepsy: report of five cases. Neurosurgery 2004;54:1395–402 [discussion: 1402–4].

33. Quigg M, Broshek DK, Barbaro NM, et al. Neuropsychological outcomes after Gamma Knife radiosurgery for mesial temporal lobe epilepsy: a prospective multicenter study. Epilepsia 2011;52:909–16.

34. Hensley-Judge H, Quigg M, Barbaro NM, et al. Visual field defects after radiosurgery for mesial temporal lobe epilepsy. Epilepsia 2013;54:1376–80.

35. Usami K, Kawai K, Koga T, et al. Delayed complication after Gamma Knife surgery for mesial temporal lobe epilepsy. J Neurosurg 2012;116:1221–5.

36. Shamisa A, Bance M, Nag S, et al. Glioblastoma multiforme occurring in a patient treated with gamma knife surgery. Case report and review of the literature. J Neurosurg 2001;94:816–21.

37. Kaido T, Hoshida T, Uranishi R, et al. Radiosurgery-induced brain tumor. Case report. J Neurosurg 2001;95:710–3.

38. Ganz JC. Gamma knife radiosurgery and its possible relationship to malignancy: a review. J Neurosurg 2002;97:644–52.

39. Quigg M, Rolston J, Barbaro NM. Radiosurgery for epilepsy: clinical experience and potential antiepileptic mechanisms. Epilepsia 2012;53:7–15.

40. Yen DJ, Chung WY, Shih YH, et al. Gamma knife radiosurgery for the treatment of recurrent seizures after incomplete anterior temporal lobectomy. Seizure 2009;18:511–4.

41. Kawai K, Suzuki I, Kurita H, et al. Failure of low-dose radiosurgery to control temporal lobe epilepsy. J Neurosurg 2001;95:883–7.

42. Cmelak AJ, Abou-Khalil B, Konrad PE, et al. Low-dose stereotactic radiosurgery is inadequate for medically intractable mesial temporal lobe epilepsy: a case report. Seizure 2001;10:442–6.

43. Regis J, Peragui JC, Rey M, et al. First selective amygdalohippocampal radiosurgery for 'mesial temporal lobe epilepsy'. Stereotact Funct Neurosurg 1995;64(Suppl 1):193–201.

44. Regis J, Bartolomei F. Comment on: failure of gamma knife radiosurgery for mesial temporal lobe epilepsy: report of five cases. Neurosurgery 2004;54:1404.

45. Regis J, Bartolomei F, Rey M, et al. Gamma knife surgery for mesial temporal lobe epilepsy. Epilepsia 1999;40:1551–6.

46. Chang EF, Quigg M, Oh MC, et al. Predictors of efficacy after stereotactic radiosurgery for medial temporal lobe epilepsy. Neurology 2010;74:165–72.

47. Yu JS, Yong WH, Wilson D, et al. Glioblastoma induction after radiosurgery for meningioma. Lancet 2000;356:1576–7.

The Stereo-Electroencephalography Methodology

Soha Alomar, MD, MPH, Jaes Jones, BS,
Andres Maldonado, MD, Jorge Gonzalez-Martinez, MD, PhD*

KEYWORDS

- Epilepsy surgery • Stereo-electroencephalography • Stereotaxy • Morbidity • Seizure outcome

KEY POINTS

- Stereo-electroencephalography (SEEG) defines the anatomic boundaries of the cortical and subcortical brain areas responsible for primary generations and early propagation of the epileptiform activity.
- Both frame-based and frameless techniques can be used for implantation of SEEG electrodes.
- Vascular imaging is fundamental for the safe implantation of SEEG electrodes. Attention to the vascular anatomy is essential to reduce the risk of hemorrhagic complications.

INTRODUCTION

One of the main goals of epilepsy surgery is the complete resection (or complete disconnection) of the cortical areas responsible for the primary organization of the epileptogenic activity. This area is also known as the epileptogenic zone (EZ). Because the EZ can eventually overlap with functional cortical areas (eloquent cortex), preservation of these necessary brain functions is another goal of any surgical resection in patients with medically refractory epilepsy.[1–7]

Because successful resective epilepsy surgery relies on accurate preoperative localization of the EZ, a preoperative evaluation is necessary to obtain the widest and most accurate spectrum of information from clinical, anatomic, and neurophysiologic aspects, with the ultimate goal of performing an individualized resection for each patient. The noninvasive methods of seizure localization and lateralization (scalp electroencephalography [EEG], imaging, magnetoencephalographic [MEG], etc) are complementary and results are interpreted in conjunction, in the attempt to compose a localization hypothesis of

the anatomic location of the EZ. When the noninvasive data are insufficient to define the EZ, extraoperative invasive monitoring may be indicated. Stereo-electroencephalography (SEEG) is among the extraoperative invasive methods that can be applied in patients with medically refractory focal epilepsy to define anatomically the EZ and the possibly related functional cortical areas. Clinical aspects of the SEEG method and technique are discussed in this article.

HISTORY AND BASIC PRINCIPLES RELATED TO THE STEREO-ELECTROENCEPHALOGRAPHY METHODOLOGY

The SEEG method was originally developed by Jean Talairach and Jean Bancaud during the 1950s[8] and has been mostly used in France, and later in Italy, as the method of choice for invasive mapping in refractory focal epilepsy.[7,9–31] In France, after the development of the stereotactic techniques and frames, which were applied initially for abnormal movement disorder surgery, Jean Talairach devoted most of his activity to the field of epilepsy. Bancaud joined

Department of Neurosurgery, Epilepsy Center, Neurological Institute, Cleveland Clinic, 9500 Euclid Avenue, Cleveland, OH 44195, USA
* Corresponding author.
E-mail address: gonzalj1@ccf.org

Neurosurg Clin N Am 27 (2016) 83–95
http://dx.doi.org/10.1016/j.nec.2015.08.003
1042-3680/16/$ – see front matter © 2016 Elsevier Inc. All rights reserved.

Talairach in 1952. The new methodology created by both physicians led them to depart very quickly from another approach that was limited to the superficial cortex. Wilder Penfield and colleagues at the Montreal Neurologic Institute did likewise. Talairach's innovative thinking was to implement a working methodology for a comprehensive analysis of morphologic and functional cerebral space. His atlas on the telencephalon, published in 1967, perfectly illustrates the new anatomic concepts for stereotaxis.[32] The development of tools, adapted to a new stereotactic frame designed by Talairach and colleagues,[32] allowed the Saint Anne investigators (Talairach and Bancaud) to propose the functional exploration of the brain by depth electrodes, allowing the exploration of both superficial and deep cortical areas. The debut of SEEG was in 1957, when the first implantation of intracerebral electrodes for epilepsy was performed on May 3 in Saint Anne Hospital (Paris, France). By departing from the then current methods of invasive monitoring, such implantations allowed for the exploration of the activity of different brain structures and for the recording of the patients' spontaneous seizures. This development was something that Penfield's method of investigation failed to achieve. In 1962, Talairach's and Bancaud's new technique and method was called "the Stereo-Electro-Encephalography."[11]

The principles of SEEG methodology remain similar to the principles originally described by Bancaud and Talairach, which are based on anatomoelectroclinical correlations (AEC) with the main aim to conceptualize the 3-dimensional (3D) spatial–temporal organization of the epileptic discharge within the brain.[7,11–13,22–31,33,34] The implantation strategy is individualized, with electrode placement based on preimplantation hypotheses that takes into consideration patient's seizures' electroclinical correlations and their relation with a suspected lesion. For these reasons, the preimplantation AEC hypotheses formulation is the single most important element in the process of planning the placement of SEEG electrodes. If the preimplantation hypotheses are incorrect, the placement of the depth electrodes will be inadequate and the interpretation of the SEEG recordings will not give access to the definition of the EZ.

CHOOSING STEREO-ELECTROENCEPHALOGRAPHY AS THE APPROPRIATE METHOD FOR EXTRAOPERATIVE INVASIVE MONITORING

After the establishment of the diagnosis of pharmacoresistant epilepsy (defined as a failure to respond to ≥2 adequately chosen and used antiepileptic medications),[35] a preoperative evaluation is indicated with 2 main goals: (1) mapping of the AEC network leading to the identification of the EZ and its extent, and (2) assessment of the functional status of the epileptogenic region(s). Achievement of both goals will lead to optimization of postresection seizure and functional outcomes. As briefly discussed, multiple techniques may be used to achieve the stated goals. Scalp video EEG monitoring is needed to confirm the diagnosis of focal epilepsy (including interictal and ictal EEG recordings) and to identify the cortical structure of the hypothetical networks that may be involved in seizure organization (through analysis of the recorded clinical and electrical semiology). Data obtained via scalp video EEG monitoring may lead to the formulation of clear AEC hypotheses. Further validation of the anatomic hypothesis is achieved through structural imaging (the identification of lesion on MRI), with or without metabolic imaging (including fluorodeoxyglucose–PET hypometabolism that may point to focal regions of cortical dysfunction). Other studies may include ictal single photon emission computed tomography, MEG, and EEG-functional MRI.[6,36,37]

These noninvasive studies identify the EZ in more than one-half of patients undergoing preoperative workup (around 70% of the patients who are operated on at Cleveland Clinic in 2012; unpublished data) Unfortunately, a formulation of a clear and unique AEC hypothesis may not be possible in the remaining 30% of patients. In such a case, focal or focal/regional epilepsy is likely, but the noninvasive phase I cannot enable caregivers to decide between 2 or 3 hypotheses in the same hemisphere. Alternatively, there is a sound regional hypothesis but not enough argument in favor of 1 hemisphere or hypotheses are generated but the exact location of the EZ, its extent, and/or its overlap with functional (eloquent) cortex remain unclear. Consequently, these patients may be candidates for an invasive evaluation using intraoperative electrocorticography or extraoperative methods such as subdural grids/strips, subdural grids combined with depth electrodes, and SEEG.[38]

In summary, the primary indications for an invasive evaluation in focal pharmacoresistant epilepsy (with the main purpose of direct cortical recording) are to address the main challenges and limitations of various noninvasive techniques. Based on the limitations outlined of the various noninvasive techniques, an invasive evaluation should be considered in any 1 of the following cases.

1. *MRI-negative cases:* The MRI does not show a cortical lesion in a location that is concordant with the electroclinical/functional hypothesis generated by the video EEG recordings.
2. *Electroclinical and MRI data discordance:* The anatomic location of the MRI identified lesion (and at times the location of a clearly hypometabolic focal area on PET) is not concordant with the electroclinical hypothesis. These include cases of deeply seated brain lesions such periventricular nodular heterotopia or deep sulcal lesions. In addition, scalp EEG recordings in 85% to 100% of patients with focal cortical dysplasia show interictal spikes that range in their distribution from lobar to lateralized, from difficult to localize to diffuse (including generalized spike-wave patterns in some cases of subependymal heterotopia).[26,27,31,39–41] The spatial distribution of interictal spikes is usually more extensive than the structural abnormality as assessed by intraoperative inspection or MRI visual analysis.[42]
3. *Multiple, in part discordant lesions:* There are 2 or more anatomic lesions with the location of at least 1 of them being discordant with the electroclinical hypothesis, or both lesions are located within the same functional network and it is unclear if 1 (or both) of them is (are) epileptic.
4. *Overlap with eloquent cortex:* The generated anatomoelectroclinical hypothesis (MRI-negative or MRI-identifiable lesion) involves potentially highly eloquent cortex. The identification of the EZ, mapping of its extent, and/or its relationship with potentially eloquent cortex are not typically resolved in these cases. These include patients with suspected focal cortical dysplasia as the possible pathologic substrate for epilepsy.[4,34,40,42–46]

In these instances, an invasive evaluation usually leads to the formulation of a clear resective surgical strategy. The recommendation for invasive monitoring and its type is made during a multidisciplinary patient management meeting that includes neurologists, neurosurgeons, neuroradiologists and neuropsychologists. Areas and networks of coverage/sampling are determined based on a well-formulated AEC hypothesis, including results of the noninvasive studies.

There is no clear consensus on the best selection criteria for each method. Some epilepsy centers have applied both technical procedures in a systematic matter, but none of them have conducted definitive comparative studies. The "pro-SEEG groups" believe this method can provide the same answers as any and all other invasive methods.[7,9–31,33,34,38,39,47–68] On the contrary, the "pro-subdural groups," who are not familiar with depth electrode explorations, tend to limit its indications strictly to the exploration of deep structures, for example, to distinguish unilateral or bilateral lobe epilepsy, and possibly to study epilepsy related to nodular heterotopia. However, differences between SEEG and subdural grids and strips are more extensive and complex than just the dichotomy between deep versus superficial mapping. The "philosophy," "definitions," and "concepts" of the 2 types of explorations are different and at times divergent. Subdural explorations were oriented initially toward the invasive study of lesional epilepsy, whereas SEEG initially takes little into account of the lesion itself. We may speculate that SEEG is more suitable to explore patients with nonlesional MRIs for whom, in some cases, it is not at all clear that surgery should be performed.[38,60–62] In addition, SEEG allows one to explore remote and multilobar areas without the need of craniotomies and the need for immediate surgery, allowing a prolonged reflection time for the patient and, consequently, a more complete informed consent process. The use and analysis of direct electrical stimulation in 1 method and the other is quite different, even opposite.[69]

Extraoperative mapping with the subdural method (including grids, strips, and the possible combination with depth electrodes) has the advantage of allowing an optimal anatomic and contiguous coverage and sampling of the adjacent cortex leading to accurate superficial cortex functional mapping exploration.[70,71] This is especially the case when there is the need to determine the extension of the EZ associated with a superficial lesion and its anatomic relation to a close functional area. This is not true if the lesion includes a deep-seated component where functional mapping cannot be obtained from subdural mapping. From a surgical perspective, subdural implantations are open procedures, with better management of occasional intracranial hemorrhagic complications. The main disadvantages of the subdural method are related to the inability to record and map deep structures such as the insular cortex, orbitofrontal cortex, cingulate gyrus, depths of sulci, and so on, and consequently, its incapacity to figure out the spatiotemporal dynamics of the epileptogenic network. In these scenarios, the SEEG methodology may be considered a more appropriate and safer option. SEEG has the advantages of allowing extensive and precise deep brain recordings and stimulations (to localize seizure onset) with minimal associated morbidity.[34,54,55,60–62]

Consequently, based on the potential advantages and disadvantages from each method, one can consider possible specific indications to choose SEEG in contrast with other methods of invasive monitoring:

1. The possibility of a deep-seated or difficult to cover location of the EZ in areas, such as the mesial structures of the temporal lobe, perisylvian areas, cingulate gyrus, and mesial interhemispheric regions, ventromedial prefrontal areas, insula, and depths of sulci.
2. A failure of a previous subdural invasive study to outline clearly the exact location of the seizure onset zone. The failure to identify the EZ in these patients may be owing to multiple reasons that include the lack of adequate sampling from a deep focus or a clinically silent focus upstream from the EZ.
3. The need for extensive, bihemispheric explorations (in particular in focal epilepsies arising from the interhemispheric or deep insular regions, or temporoparietooccipital junction).
4. Preoperative evaluation suggestive of extended network involvement (eg, temporofrontal or frontoparietal) in the setting of a normal MRI (**Table 1**).

A majority of patients undergoing reoperations may have failed epilepsy surgery during preceding subdural evaluations because of difficulties in accurately localizing the EZ. These patients pose a significant dilemma for further management, having relatively few options available. Further open subdural grid evaluations may carry the risks associated with encountering scar formations, and still having limitations related to deep cortical structure recordings. A subsequent evaluation using the SEEG method may overcome these limitations, offering an additional opportunity for seizure localization and sustained seizure freedom.[54] The hypothetical disadvantage of the SEEG method is the more restricted capability for performing functional mapping. Owing to the limited number of contacts located in the superficial cortex, a contiguous mapping of eloquent brain areas cannot be obtained, as in the subdural mapping method.[34,54,55] Functional mapping in SEEG cannot be dissociated from the electroclinical localization process and, consequently, a fair comparison between both methods cannot be performed. In addition, the precision of the subdural functional mapping is far from being validated. Last, the functional mapping information extracted from the SEEG method can be complemented frequently with other methods of mapping, such as diffusion tensor images or awake craniotomies,[34] diminishing the relative disadvantages claimed by the "subdural groups."

HOW TO SELECT THE STEREO-ELECTROENCEPHALOGRAPHY TRAJECTORIES: PLANNING THE IMPLANTATION

As indicated, the development of an SEEG implantation plan requires the clear formulation of precise AEC hypotheses to be tested. These hypotheses are typically generated during the multidisciplinary patient management conference based on the results of various noninvasive tests. At the Cleveland Clinic, a final tailored implantation strategy is generated during a separate preoperative

Table 1
Selection criteria for different methods of invasive monitoring in medically refractory focal epilepsy

Clinical Scenario	Method of Choice	Second Option
Lesional MRI: Potential epileptogenic lesion is superficially located, near or in the proximity of eloquent cortex. Nonlesional MRI: Hypothetical EZ located in the proximity of eloquent cortex.	SDG	SEEG
Lesional MRI: Potential epileptogenic lesion is located in deep cortical and subcortical areas. Nonlesional MRI: hypothetical EZ is deeply located or located in noneloquent areas.	SEEG	SDG with depths
Need for bilateral explorations and or reoperations.	SEEG	SDG with depths
After subdural grids failure	SEEG	SDG with depths
When the AEC hypothesis suggest the involvement of a more extensive, multilobar epileptic network.	SEEG	SDG with depths
Suspected frontal lobe epilepsy in nonlesional MRI scenario	SEEG	SEEG

Abbreviations: AEC, anatomoelectroclinical correlations; EZ, epileptogenic zone; SDG, subdural grid; SEEG, Stereo-electroencephalography.

implantation meeting. Depth electrodes should sample the anatomic lesion (if identified), the more likely structure(s) of ictal onset, the early and late spread regions, and the interactions with the functional (cognitive, sensorimotor, behavioral, etc.) networks. A 3D "conceptualization" of the network nodes upstream and downstream from the hypothesized epileptogenic network is an essential component of the preoperative implantation strategy. Initially, by analyzing the available noninvasive data and the temporal evolution of the ictal clinical manifestations, a hypothesis of the anatomic location of the EZ is formulated.[72] The implantation plan is created in collaboration with experienced epileptologists, neurosurgeons, and neuroradiologists who together formulate hypotheses for EZ localization. Adequate knowledge of the possible functional networks involved in the primary organization of the epileptic activity is mandatory to formulate accurate hypotheses. In addition, the treating physicians will have to take into account the 3D aspects of depth electrode recordings that, despite a limited coverage (which is largely compensated by the interpolation process made possible by the electrophysiologic methodology—namely, frequencies, spatial relations, and latencies analyses) of the cortical surface compared with subdural grids and strips, enable an accurate sampling of the structures along its trajectory, from the entry site to the final impact point. Therefore, the trajectory is more important than the target or entry point areas. Consequently, the investigation may include lateral and mesial surfaces of the different lobes, deep-seated cortices such as the depths of sulci, insula, posterior areas in the interhemispheric cortical surface, and so on. The implantation should also consider the different cortical cytoarchitectonic areas involved in seizure organization patterns and their likely connectivity to other cortical and subcortical areas. It is important to emphasize that the implantation strategy focus is not to map lobes or lobules, but epileptogenic networks that, in general, involve multiple lobes. Furthermore, exploration strategy should also take into consideration possible alternative hypotheses of localization.[57,62,73]

Last, the aim to obtain all the possible information from the SEEG exploration should not be pursued at the expenses of an excessive number of electrodes, which will likely increase the morbidity of the implantation. In general, implantations that exceed 15 depth electrodes are rare. In addition, the possible involvement of eloquent regions in the ictal discharge requires their judicious coverage, with the 2-fold goal to assess their role in the seizure organization and to define the boundaries of a safe surgical resection (**Fig. 1**).

The SEEG implantation patterns are based on a tailored strategy of exploration, which results from the primary hypothesis of the anatomic location of the EZ, for every single case. As a consequence, standard implantations for specific areas and lobes are difficult to conceptualize. Nevertheless, a number of typical patterns of coverage can be recognized.

Limbic Network Explorations

Cases of temporal lobe epilepsy with consistent anatomoelectroclinical findings suggesting a limbic network involvement are usually operated on after noninvasive investigation only. In general, the use of invasive monitoring is not necessary when semiological and electrophysiologic studies demonstrate typical nondominant mesial temporal epilepsy and imaging studies shows a clear lesion (mesial temporal sclerosis, as an example) that fits the initial localization hypothesis. Nevertheless, invasive exploration with SEEG recordings may be required in patients in whom the supposed EZs, probably involving the temporal lobes, are suspected to involve extratemporal areas as well. In these cases, the implantation pattern points to disclose a preferential spread of the discharge to the temporoinsular anterior perisylvian areas, the temporoinsular orbitofrontal areas, or the posterior temporal, posterior insula, temporobasal, parietal, and posterior cingulate areas. Consequently, sampling of extratemporal limbic areas must be wide enough to provide information to identify a possible extratemporal origin of the seizures that could not been anticipated with precision according to noninvasive methods of investigation.

Frontal–Parietal Network Explorations

Owing to the large volume of the frontal and parietal lobes, a high number of electrodes are required for an adequate coverage of this region. In most patients, however, excessive sampling can be avoided, and the implantation to more limited portions of the frontal and parietal lobes can be performed. The suspicion of orbitofrontal epilepsy, for instance, often requires the investigation of the gyrus rectus, the frontal polar areas, the anterior cingulate gyrus, and the anterior portions of the temporal lobe (temporal pole). Similarly, seizures that are thought to arise from the mesial wall of the premotor cortex are evaluated by targeting at least the rostral and caudal part of the supplementary motor area, the pre–supplementary motor area, different portions of the cingulate gyrus and sulcus, as well as the primary motor

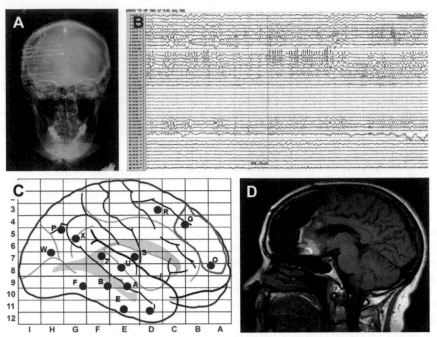

Fig. 1. A 65-year-old female patient with intractable epilepsy and nonlesional MRI. (*A*) Anteroposterior (AP) x-ray showing right stereo-electroencephalography implantation. (*B*) Interictal spikes from the right mesial frontal electrode. (*C*) Ictal onset from right mesial frontal electrode (G) and right frontopolar electrode (O). (*D*) Postoperative MRI showing right frontal resection of G and O electrode regions as well as the nonsampled orbitofrontal region.

cortex and mesial and dorsal–lateral parietal cortex. Consequently, the hypothesis-based sampling often allows localization of the EZ in the frontal and/or parietal lobes, and in some cases may allow the identification of relatively small EZs. Occasionally, frontal–parietal network explorations may be bilateral, and sometimes symmetric, mainly when a mesial frontal–parietal epilepsy is suspected and the noninvasive methods of investigation failed in lateralizing the epileptic activity.

Electrodes in rolandic regions are normally placed when there is a need to define the posterior margin of the resection in frontal network explorations or the anterior margin in parietal–occipital explorations, or when the EZ may be located in or near rolandic cortex. The main goal here is to evaluate the rolandic participation to the ictal discharge and to obtain a functional mapping by intracerebral electrical stimulation. In this location, depth electrodes are particularly helpful to sample the depth of the central sulcus, as well as the descending and ascending white matter fibers associated with this region.

Posterior Quadrant Network Explorations

In the posterior quadrant, placement of electrodes limited to a single lobe is extremely uncommon,

owing to the frequent simultaneous involvement of several occipital, parietal, and posterior temporal structures, as well as to the multidirectional spread of the discharges to suprasylvian and infrasylvian areas. Consequently, mesial and dorsal lateral surfaces of the occipital lobes are explored, covering both infracalcarine and supracalcarine areas, in association with posterior temporal, posterior perisylvian, basal temporal–occipital areas, and posterior parietal areas including the posterior inferior parietal lobule and the posterior precuneus. In posterior quadrant epilepsies, bilateral explorations are generally needed owing to rapid contralateral spread of ictal activity.

"NUTS AND BOLTS" OF THE STEREO-ELECTROENCEPHALOGRAPHY IMPLANTATION TECHNIQUE

Once the SEEG planning is finalized, the desired targets are reached using commercially available depth electrodes in various lengths and number of contacts, depending on the specific brain regions to be explored. The depth electrodes are implanted using conventional stereotactic technique or by the assistance of stereotactic robotic devices through 2.5-mm diameter drill holes. In both techniques, depth electrodes are inserted through 2.5-mm diameter drill holes, using orthogonal or oblique orientation, allowing intracranial recording from lateral, intermediate or deep cortical and subcortical structures in a 3D arrangement, thus accounting for the dynamic, multidirectional spatiotemporal organization of the epileptogenic pathways.

Initially, frame-based implantations were performed in our center. As part of our routine practice, patients were admitted to the hospital on the day of surgery. The day before surgery, a stereo contrasted volumetric T1 sequence MRI was performed. Images were then transferred to our stereotactic neuronavigation software (iPlan Cranial 2.6, Brainlab AG, Feldkirchen, Germany) where trajectories were planned the following day. The day of surgery, while the patients were under general anesthesia, Leksell stereotactic frames (Elekta, Stockholm, Sweden) were applied using the standard technique. Once the patients were attached to the angiography table with the frame, stereo dyna CT and 3D digital subtracted angiogram were performed. The preoperative MRI, the stereo dyna CT, and angiographic images were then processed digitally using a dedicated fusion software (Syngo XWP, Siemens Healthcare, Forchheim, Germany). These fused images were used during the implantation procedure to confirm the accuracy of the final position of each electrode and to insure the absence of vascular structures along the electrode pathway, which might not be noted on contrasted MRI images (**Fig. 2**). After the planning phase using the stereotactic software, trajectories' coordinates were recorded and transported to the operating room. Trajectories were, in general, planned in orthogonal orientation in relation to the skull's sagittal plane to facilitate implantation and interpretation of the electrode positions and recordings. Using the Leksell stereotactic system, coordinates for each trajectory were then adjusted in the frame and a lateral view fluoroscopic image was performed in each new position. Care was taken to ensure that the central beam of radiation during fluoroscopy was centered in the middle of the implantation probe to avoid parallax errors. If the trajectory was aligned correctly, corresponding to the planned trajectory and passing along an avascular space, the implantation was then continued, with skull perforation, dura opening, placement of the guiding bolt, and final insertion of the electrode under fluoroscopic guidance. By fusing the preimplantation angiogram with the live fluoroscopy images, a possible vessel collision could be predicted and the trajectory adjusted accordingly. If a vessel was recognized along the pathway during fluoroscopy, the guiding tube was moved manually a few millimeters until the next avascular space was recognized and implantation was then continued. The electrode insertion progress was observed under live fluoroscopic control in a frontal view to confirm the straight trajectory of each electrode. For additional guidance, a coronal MRI slice corresponding with the level of each electrode implantation was overlaid onto the fluoroscopic image.

Postimplantation dynaCT scans were performed while the patients were still anesthetized and positioned on the operating table. The reconstructed images were then fused with the MRI dataset using the previously described fusion software. The resulting merged datasets were displayed and reviewed in axial, sagittal and coronal planes allowing verification of the correct placement of the depth electrodes.[62]

More recently, robotic-assisted devices were applied. Similar to the conventional approach, volumetric preoperative MRIs are obtained and DICOM format images are digitally transferred to the robot's native planning software. Individual trajectories are planned within the 3D imaging reconstruction according to predetermined target locations and intended trajectories. Trajectories are selected to maximize sampling from superficial and deep cortical and subcortical areas within the preselected zones of interest and are oriented orthogonally in the majority of cases to facilitate the anatomoelectrophysiologic correlation during the extraoperative recording phase and to avoid possible trajectory shifts owing to excessively angled entry points. Nevertheless, when multiple targets are potentially accessible via a single nonorthogonal trajectory, these multitarget trajectories are selected to minimize the number of implanted electrodes per patient.

All trajectories are evaluated for safety and target accuracy in their individually reconstructed planes (axial, sagittal, coronal), and also along the reconstructed "probe's eye view." Any trajectories that seem to compromise vascular structures are adjusted appropriately without affecting the sampling from areas of interest. A set working distance of 150 mm from the drilling platform to the target is used initially for each trajectory, being later adjusted to maximally reduce the working distance and, consequently, improve the accuracy of the implantation. The overall implantation schemas are analyzed using the 3D cranial reconstruction capabilities. Internal trajectories are checked to ensure that no trajectory collisions are present. External trajectory positions are examined for any entry sites that would be prohibitively close (<1.5 cm distance) at the skin level.

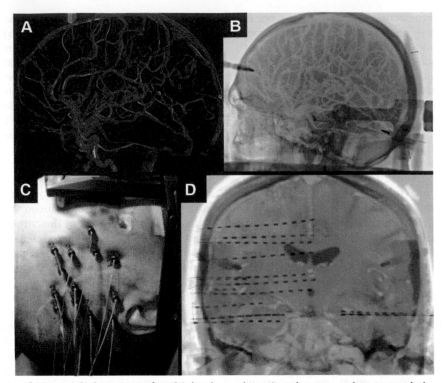

Fig. 2. Imaging fusion and placement of multiple electrodes using the stereo-electroencephalography (SEEG) method. (*A, B*) Preoperative imaging with MR angiography and angiography, respectively. Together, electrode trajectories are safely planned, avoiding vascular structures, and limiting the risk of bleeding and electrode misplacement. (*C*) Fourteen electrodes at the skin surface. (*D*) Intraoperative image showing a superposition of bilateral SEEG electrodes on a coronal MRI T1-weighted image. Note the precise parallel placement, with tips terminating at the midline or dural surface.

On the day of surgery, patients are placed under general anesthesia. For each patient, the head is placed into a 3-point fixation head holder. The robot is then positioned such that the working distance (distance between the base of the robotic arm and the midpoint of the cranium) is approximately 70 cm. The robot is locked into position, and the head holder device is secured to the robot. No additional position adjustments are made to the operating table during the implantation procedure. After positioning and securing the patient to the robot, image registrations are performed. Semiautomatic laser based facial recognition is used to register the preoperative volumetric MRI with the patient. The laser is first calibrated using a set distance calibration tool. Preset anatomic facial landmarks are then selected manually with the laser. The areas defined by the manually entered anatomic landmarks subsequently undergo automatic registration using laser-based facial surface scanning. The accuracy of the registration process is then confirmed by correlating additional, independently chosen surface landmarks with the registered MRI. After successful registration, the planned trajectories'

accessibilities are automatically verified by the robot software.

The patients are then prepped and draped in a standard sterile fashion. The robotic working arm is also draped with a sterile plastic cover. A drilling platform, with a 2.5-mm diameter working cannula, is secured to the robotic arm. The desired trajectories are selected on the touch screen interface. After trajectory confirmation, the arm movement is initiated through the use of a foot pedal. The robotic arm automatically locks the drilling platform into a stable position once the calculated position for the selected trajectory is reached. A 2-mm diameter handheld drill (Stryker, Kalamazoo, MI) is introduced through the platform and used to create a pinhole. The dura is then opened with an insulated dural perforator using monopolar cautery at low settings. A guiding bolt (Ad-Tech, Racine, WI) is screwed firmly into each pinhole. The distance from the drilling platform to the retaining bolt is measured and this value is subtracted from the standardized 150-mm platform to target distance. The resulting difference is recorded for later use as the final length of the electrode to be implanted. This process is repeated for each trajectory. All pinholes and retaining bolts are placed before the electrode insertions, for both orthogonal and angled trajectories. Once the guiding bolts are implanted in specific angles of insertion, no additional trajectory modifications are performed. Subsequently, for each trajectory, a small stylet (1 mm in diameter) is then set to the previously recorded electrode distance and passed gently into the parenchyma, guided by the implantation bolt, followed immediately by the insertion of the premeasured electrode (**Figs. 3** and **4**).

MORBIDITY AND SEIZURE OUTCOME

Our center recently reported 200 patients undergoing 2663 SEEG electrode implantations for the purposes of invasive intracranial EEG monitoring, in accordance with a tailored preimplantation hypothesis to investigate and anatomically characterize the extension of the EZ. The studied group was challenging owing to the paucity of noninvasive data and/or the possibility of a more diffuse pathology suggested by a previous failure invasive monitoring exploration; nearly one-third of the

studied patients (58 patients [29%]) were individuals who had undergone prior surgical intervention for medically refractory epilepsy, resulting in postoperative recurrent seizures. Despite the challenging and discourage clinical scenario, the SEEG method was able to confirm the EZ in 154 patients (77.0%). Of these, 134 patients (87.0%) underwent subsequent craniotomy for SEEG guided resection. Within this cohort, 90 patients had a minimum postoperative follow-up of at least 12 months; therein, 61 patients (67.8%) remained seizure free (ie, Engel I outcome). The most common pathologic diagnosis in this group was focal cortical dysplasia type I (55 patients; 61.1%). Complications were minimal. They included wound infections (0.08%), hemorrhagic complications (0.08%), and a transient neurologic deficit (0.04%) in a total of 5 patients. The total morbidity rate was 2.5%.

Results in terms of seizure outcome and complications are compatible with already published results from other groups. These results parallel those of previous studies in the recent literature. Munari and colleagues[74] (1994) reported on their experience with SEEG in 70 patients undergoing

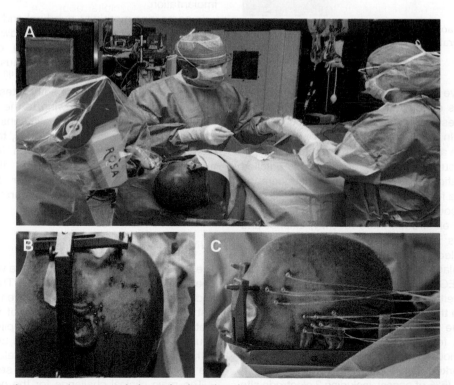

Fig. 3. Robotic stereo-electroencephalography (SEEG) technique. (*A*) Operating room "set up" during left side SEEG robotic implantation, with surgeon and scrub nurse positioned on each side of the patient, and the robot device placed approximately 150 mm from the center of the patient's head, in the middle, at the vertex. (*B*) Intraoperative aspect of left side frontal–temporal SEEG implantation with the guiding bolts in their final position. (*C*) Left side frontal–temporal SEEG implantation after the implantation of depth electrodes. Final aspect.

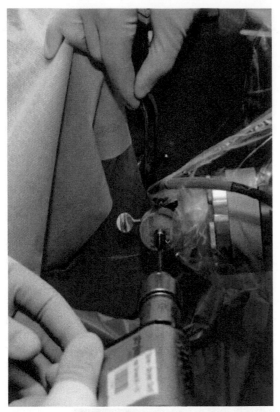

Fig. 4. Intraoperative picture showing the drilling of a left temporal trajectory guided by the robotic device.

a collective total of 712 electrode implantations. Within this cohort, an individualized and tailored surgical resection was performed in 60 patients (85.7%). In their series, specifically relating to SEEG, the authors identified 1 permanent complication ensuing from the procedure; this entailed the formation of an asymptomatic intracerebral hematoma following the removal of an SEEG electrode (accounting for a morbidity rate of 1.4%, or 0.1% per electrode). More recently, Guenot and colleagues[75] (2001) presented a series of 100 patients collectively undergoing 1118 SEEG electrode implantations for invasive EEG monitoring. Here, SEEG was deemed helpful in 84 patients (84%) by either annulling or confirming (and additionally, in the latter case, guiding) surgical resection of the EZ. Moreover, SEEG confirmed the indication for resection in 14 cases (14%) that were previously disputed on the basis of the noninvasive workup. These authors reported on 5 complications (5% of cases), including 2 electrode site infections (0.2% per electrode), 2 intracranial electrode fractures (0.2% per electrode), and 1 intracerebral hematoma resulting in death (accounting for a mortality rate of 1% in the study). In a large

series, Cossu and colleagues[76] reported a morbidity rate of 5.6%, with severe permanent deficits from intracerebral hemorrhage in 1%. In another study, Tanriverdi and colleagues[77] (2009) summarized their experience with a subgroup of 491 refractory epilepsy patients collectively undergoing 2490 intracerebral SEEG electrode implantations and 2943 depth electrode implantations.[77] Based on the authors' experience, they identified 4 patients (0.8%) with an intracranial hematoma at the electrode site (0.07% per electrode) and 9 patients (1.8%) with an infection arising from electrode placement (0.2% per electrode); moreover, they reported no mortalities ensuing directly from SEEG electrode placement. Finally, Cardinale and colleagues[73] (2013) most recently presented their experience with 6496 electrodes stereotactically implanted in 482 epilepsy patients with refractory epilepsy. These authors identified 2 patients (0.4%, or 0.03% per electrode) with permanent neurologic deficits in their series; 14 patients (2.9%, or 0.2% per electrode) with hemorrhagic complication; 2 patients (0.4%, or 0.03% per electrode) with infection; and 1 mortality (0.2%) resulting from massive brain edema and concomitant hyponatremia after electrode implantation.

In comparing morbidity, subdural grid electrode implantation has historically been shown to have low permanent morbidity (0%–3%) compared with depth electrodes (3%–6%) because there is no intraparenchymal passage.[2,37,78–83] Although it is difficult to compare morbidity rates between subdural grids and SEEG owing to the variability in patient selection, different institutions and variable number of implanted electrodes, the clinical experience among different groups in Europe and North America suggests that the SEEG method provides at least a similar degree of safety when compared with subdural grids or strips.[7,28,29,33,38,57,61,64,74,77,83–86]

SUMMARY

The SEEG methodology and technique was developed almost 60 years ago in Europe. The efficacy and safety of SEEG has been proven over the last 55 years. The main advantage of the SEEG method is the possibility to study the epileptogenic neuronal network in its dynamic and 3D aspect, with an optimal time and space correlation, with the clinical semiology of the patient's seizures.

The main clinical challenge for the near future remains in the further refinement of specific selection criteria for the different methods of invasive monitoring, with the ultimate goal of comparing and validating the results (long-term seizure-free outcome) obtained from different methods of invasive monitoring.

REFERENCES

1. Rosenow F, Luders H. Presurgical evaluation of epilepsy. Brain 2001;124(Pt 9):1683–700.
2. Wyllie E, Luders H, Morris HH 3rd, et al. Subdural electrodes in the evaluation for epilepsy surgery in children and adults. Neuropediatrics 1988;19(2):80–6.
3. Jayakar P, Duchowny M, Resnick TJ. Subdural monitoring in the evaluation of children for epilepsy surgery. J Child Neurol 1994;9(Suppl 2):61–6.
4. Adelson PD, O'Rourke DK, Albright AL. Chronic invasive monitoring for identifying seizure foci in children. Neurosurg Clin N Am 1995;6(3):491–504.
5. Jayakar P. Invasive EEG monitoring in children: when, where, and what? J Clin Neurophysiol 1999; 16(5):408–18.
6. Winkler PA, Herzog C, Henkel A, et al. Noninvasive protocol for surgical treatment of focal epilepsies. Nervenarzt 1999;70(12):1088–93 [in German].
7. Cossu M, Chabardes S, Hoffmann D, et al. Presurgical evaluation of intractable epilepsy using stereo-electro-encephalography methodology: principles, technique and morbidity. Neurochirurgie 2008; 54(3):367–73 [in French].
8. Bancaud J, Dell MB. Technics and method of stereotaxic functional exploration of the brain structures in man (cortex, subcortex, central gray nuclei). Rev Neurol 1959;101:213–27 [in French].
9. Bancaud J, Talairach J, Waltregny P, et al. Stimulation of focal cortical epilepsies by megimide in topographic diagnosis. (Clinical EEG and SEEG study). Rev Neurol (Paris) 1968;119(3):320–5 [in French].
10. Bancaud J, Talairach J, Waltregny P, et al. Activation by Megimide in the topographic diagnosis of focal cortical epilepsies (clinical EEG and SEEG study). Electroencephalogr Clin Neurophysiol 1969;26(6):640.
11. Bancaud J, Angelergues R, Bernouilli C, et al. Functional stereotaxic exploration (SEEG) of epilepsy. Electroencephalogr Clin Neurophysiol 1970;28(1): 85–6.
12. Bancaud J, Favel P, Bonis A, et al. Paroxysmal sexual manifestations and temporal lobe epilepsy. Clinical, EEG and SEEG study of a case of epilepsy of tumoral origin. Rev Neurol (Paris) 1970;123(4): 217–30 [in French].
13. Bancaud J, Talairach J. Methodology of stereo EEG exploration and surgical intervention in epilepsy. Rev Otoneuroophtalmol 1973;45(4):315–28 [in French].
14. Geier S, Bancaud J, Talairach J, et al. Radio-telemetry in EEG and SEEG. Technology and material. Rev Electroencephalogr Neurophysiol Clin 1973; 3(4):353–4 [in French].
15. Cabrini GP, Ettorre G, Marossero F, et al. Surgery of epilepsy: some indications for SEEG. J Neurosurg Sci 1975;19(1–2):95–104.
16. Bancaud J, Talairach J, Geier S, et al. Behavioral manifestations induced by electric stimulation of the anterior cingulate gyrus in man. Rev Neurol (Paris) 1976;132(10):705–24 [in French].
17. Musolino A, Tournoux P, Missir O, et al. Methodology of "in vivo" anatomical study and stereo-electroencephalographic exploration in brain surgery for epilepsy. J Neuroradiol 1990;17(2):67–102.
18. Engel J Jr, Henry TR, Risinger MW, et al. Presurgical evaluation for partial epilepsy: relative contributions of chronic depth-electrode recordings versus FDG-PET and scalp-sphenoidal ictal EEG. Neurology 1990;40(11):1670–7.
19. Baucaud J, Talairach J, Munari C, et al. Introduction to the clinical study of postrolandic epileptic seizures. Can J Neurol Sci 1991;18(Suppl 4):566–9 [in French].
20. Talairach J, Bancaud J, Bonis A, et al. Surgical therapy for frontal epilepsies. Adv Neurol 1992;57:707–32.
21. Avanzini G. Discussion of stereoelectroencephalography. Acta Neurol Scand Suppl 1994;152:70–3.
22. Bartolomei F, Wendling F, Bellanger JJ, et al. Neural networks involving the medial temporal structures in temporal lobe epilepsy. Clin Neurophysiol 2001; 112(9):1746–60.
23. Biraben A, Taussig D, Thomas P, et al. Fear as the main feature of epileptic seizures. J Neurol Neurosurg Psychiatry 2001;70(2):186–91.
24. Wendling F, Bartolomei F, Bellanger JJ, et al. Interpretation of interdependencies in epileptic signals using a macroscopic physiological model of the EEG. Clin Neurophysiol 2001;112(7):1201–18.
25. Wendling F, Bartolomei F, Bellanger JJ, et al. Identification of epileptogenic networks from modeling and nonlinear analysis of SEEG signals. Neurophysiol Clin 2001;31(3):139–51 [in French].
26. Tassi L, Colombo N, Cossu M, et al. Electroclinical, MRI and neuropathological study of 10 patients with nodular heterotopia, with surgical outcomes. Brain 2005;128(Pt 2):321–37.
27. Battaglia G, Chiapparini L, Franceschetti S, et al. Periventricular nodular heterotopia: classification, epileptic history, and genesis of epileptic discharges. Epilepsia 2006;47(1):86–97.
28. Cossu M, Cardinale F, Castana L, et al. Stereo-EEG in children. Childs Nerv Syst 2006;22(8):766–78.
29. Sindou M, Guenot M, Isnard J, et al. Temporo-mesial epilepsy surgery: outcome and complications in 100 consecutive adult patients. Acta Neurochir (Wien) 2006;148(1):39–45.
30. Guenot M, Isnard J. Epilepsy and insula. Neurochirurgie 2008;54(3):374–81 [in French].
31. Guenot M, Isnard J. Multiple SEEG-guided RF-thermolesions of epileptogenic foci. Neurochirurgie 2008;54(3):441–7 [in French].

32. Talairach J, Bancaud J, Bonis A, et al. Functional stereotaxic investigations in epilepsy. Methodological remarks concerning a case. Rev Neurol (Paris) 1961;105:119–30 [in French].

33. Devaux B, Chassoux F, Guenot M, et al. Epilepsy surgery in France. Neurochirurgie 2008;54(3):453–65 [in French].

34. Gonzalez-Martinez J, Bulacio J, Alexopoulos A, et al. Stereoelectroencephalography in the "difficult to localize" refractory focal epilepsy: early experience from a North American epilepsy center. Epilepsia 2013;54(2):323–30.

35. Kwan P, Brodie MJ. Definition of refractory epilepsy: defining the indefinable? Lancet Neurol 2010;9(1):27–9.

36. Najm IM, Naugle R, Busch RM, et al. Definition of the epileptogenic zone in a patient with non-lesional temporal lobe epilepsy arising from the dominant hemisphere. Epileptic Disord 2006;8(Suppl 2):S27–35.

37. Nair DR, Burgess R, McIntyre CC, et al. Chronic subdural electrodes in the management of epilepsy. Clin Neurophysiol 2008;119(1):11–28.

38. Gonzalez-Martinez J, Najm IM. Indications and selection criteria for invasive monitoring in children with cortical dysplasia. Childs Nerv Syst 2014;30(11):1823–9.

39. Marnet D, Devaux B, Chassoux F, et al. Surgical resection of focal cortical dysplasias in the central region. Neurochirurgie 2008;54(3):399–408 [in French].

40. Russo GL, Tassi L, Cossu M, et al. Focal cortical resection in malformations of cortical development. Epileptic Disord 2003;5(Suppl 2):S115–23.

41. Luders H, Schuele SU. Epilepsy surgery in patients with malformations of cortical development. Curr Opin Neurol 2006;19(2):169–74.

42. Kellinghaus C, Moddel G, Shigeto H, et al. Dissociation between in vitro and in vivo epileptogenicity in a rat model of cortical dysplasia. Epileptic Disord 2007;9(1):11–9.

43. Gonzalez-Martinez JA, Srikijvilaikul T, Nair D, et al. Long-term seizure outcome in reoperation after failure of epilepsy surgery. Neurosurgery 2007;60(5):873–80 [discussion: 873–80].

44. Tassi L, Colombo N, Garbelli R, et al. Focal cortical dysplasia: neuropathological subtypes, EEG, neuroimaging and surgical outcome. Brain 2002;125(Pt 8):1719–32.

45. Srikijvilaikul T, Najm IM, Hovinga CA, et al. Seizure outcome after temporal lobectomy in temporal lobe cortical dysplasia. Epilepsia 2003;44(11):1420–4.

46. Francione S, Kahane P, Tassi L, et al. Stereo-EEG of interictal and ictal electrical activity of a histologically proved heterotopic gray matter associated with partial epilepsy. Electroencephalogr Clin Neurophysiol 1994;90(4):284–90.

47. Catenoix H, Mauguiere F, Guenot M, et al. SEEG-guided thermocoagulations: a palliative treatment of nonoperable partial epilepsies. Neurology 2008;71(21):1719–26.

48. Abraham G, Zizzadoro C, Kacza J, et al. Growth and differentiation of primary and passaged equine bronchial epithelial cells under conventional and air-liquid-interface culture conditions. BMC Vet Res 2011;7:26.

49. Kerr MS, Burns SP, Gale J, et al. Multivariate analysis of SEEG signals during seizure. Conference proceedings. Annual International Conference of the IEEE Engineering in Medicine and Biology Society. IEEE Engineering in Medicine and Biology Society. Annual Conference. Boston, August 30 - September 03, 2011:8279–82.

50. Centeno RS, Yacubian EM, Caboclo LO, et al. Intracranial depth electrodes implantation in the era of image-guided surgery. Arq Neuropsiquiatr 2011;69(4):693–8.

51. Kakisaka Y, Kubota Y, Wang ZI, et al. Use of simultaneous depth and MEG recording may provide complementary information regarding the epileptogenic region. pileptic Disord 2012;14(3):298–303.

52. Yaffe R, Burns S, Gale J, et al. Brain state evolution during seizure and under anesthesia: a network-based analysis of stereotaxic EEG activity in drug-resistant epilepsy patients. Conference proceedings. Annual International Conference of the IEEE Engineering in Medicine and Biology Society. IEEE Engineering in Medicine and Biology Society. Annual Conference. San Diego, August 28 - September 01, 2012:5158–61.

53. Antony AR, Alexopoulos AV, Gonzalez-Martinez JA, et al. Functional connectivity estimated from intracranial EEG predicts surgical outcome in intractable temporal lobe epilepsy. PLoS One 2013;8(10):e77916.

54. Vadera S, Marathe AR, Gonzalez-Martinez J, et al. Stereoelectroencephalography for continuous two-dimensional cursor control in a brain-machine interface. Neurosurg Focus 2013;34(6):E3.

55. Vadera S, Mullin J, Bulacio J, et al. Stereoelectroencephalography following subdural grid placement for difficult to localize epilepsy. Neurosurgery 2013;72(5):723–9 [discussion: 729].

56. Wang S, Wang IZ, Bulacio JC, et al. Ripple classification helps to localize the seizure-onset zone in neocortical epilepsy. Epilepsia 2013;54(2):370–6.

57. Cardinale F, Cossu M, Castana L, et al. Stereoelectroencephalography: surgical methodology, safety, and stereotactic application accuracy in 500 procedures. Neurosurgery 2013;72(3):353–66 [discussion: 366].

58. Enatsu R, Bulacio J, Nair DR, et al. Posterior cingulate epilepsy: clinical and neurophysiological analysis. J Neurol Neurosurg Psychiatry 2014;85(1):44–50.

59. Enatsu R, Bulacio J, Najm I, et al. Combining stereo-electroencephalography and subdural electrodes in the diagnosis and treatment of medically intractable epilepsy. J Clin Neurosci 2014;21(8):1441–5.

60. Gonzalez-Martinez J, Lachhwani D. Stereoelectroencephalography in children with cortical dysplasia: technique and results. Childs Nerv Syst 2014;30(11): 1853–7.

61. Gonzalez-Martinez J, Mullin J, Bulacio J, et al. Stereoelectroencephalography in children and adolescents with difficult-to-localize refractory focal epilepsy. Neurosurgery 2014;75(3):258–68 [discussion: 267–8].

62. Gonzalez-Martinez J, Mullin J, Vadera S, et al. Stereotactic placement of depth electrodes in medically intractable epilepsy. J Neurosurg 2014; 120(3):639–44.

63. Johnson MA, Thompson S, Gonzalez-Martinez J, et al. Performing behavioral tasks in subjects with intracranial electrodes. J Vis Exp 2014;(92):e51947.

64. Serletis D, Bulacio J, Bingaman W, et al. The stereotactic approach for mapping epileptic networks: a prospective study of 200 patients. J Neurosurg 2014;121(5):1239–46.

65. Vadera S, Burgess R, Gonzalez-Martinez J. Concomitant use of stereoelectroencephalography (SEEG) and magnetoencephalographic (MEG) in the surgical treatment of refractory focal epilepsy. Clin Neurol Neurosurg 2014;122:9–11.

66. Cardinale F, Cossu M. Letter to the editor: SEEG has the lowest rate of complications. J Neurosurg 2014;1–3.

67. Cossu M, Fuschillo D, Cardinale F, et al. Stereo-EEG-guided radio-frequency thermocoagulations of epileptogenic grey-matter nodular heterotopy. J Neurol Neurosurg Psychiatry 2014;85(6):611–7.

68. Enatsu R, Gonzalez-Martinez J, Bulacio J, et al. Connections of the limbic network: a corticocortical evoked potentials study. Cortex 2015;62:20–33.

69. Kovac S, Kahane P, Diehl B. Seizures induced by direct electrical cortical stimulation - Mechanisms and clinical considerations. Clin Neurophysiol 2014. [Epub ahead of print].

70. Najm IM, Bingaman WE, Luders HO. The use of subdural grids in the management of focal malformations due to abnormal cortical development. Neurosurg Clin N Am 2002;13(1):87–92. viii-ix.

71. Widdess-Walsh P, Jeha L, Nair D, et al. Subdural electrode analysis in focal cortical dysplasia: predictors of surgical outcome. Neurology 2007;69(7): 660–7.

72. Chauvel P, McGonigal A. Emergence of semiology in epileptic seizures. Epilepsy Behav 2014;38:94–103.

73. Cardinale F, Lo Russo G. Stereo-electroencephalography safety and effectiveness: some more reasons in favor of epilepsy surgery. Epilepsia 2013;54(8): 1505–6.

74. Munari C, Hoffmann D, Francione S, et al. Stereo-electroencephalography methodology: advantages and limits. Acta Neurol Scand Suppl 1994;152: 56–67 [discussion: 68–9].

75. Guenot M, Isnard J, Ryvlin P, et al. Neurophysiological monitoring for epilepsy surgery: the Talairach SEEG method. StereoElectroEncephaloGraphy. Indications, results, complications and therapeutic applications in a series of 100 consecutive cases. Stereotact Funct Neurosurg 2001;77(1–4):29–32.

76. Cossu M, Cardinale F, Colombo N, et al. Stereoelectroencephalography in the presurgical evaluation of children with drug-resistant focal epilepsy. J Neurosurg 2005;103(Suppl 4):333–43.

77. Tanriverdi T, Ajlan A, Poulin N, et al. Morbidity in epilepsy surgery: an experience based on 2449 epilepsy surgery procedures from a single institution. J Neurosurg 2009;110(6):1111–23.

78. Lee WS, Lee JK, Lee SA, et al. Complications and results of subdural grid electrode implantation in epilepsy surgery. Surg Neurol 2000;54(5):346–51.

79. Rydenhag B, Silander HC. Complications of epilepsy surgery after 654 procedures in Sweden, September 1990-1995: a multicenter study based on the Swedish National Epilepsy Surgery Register. Neurosurgery 2001;49(1):51–6 [discussion: 56–7].

80. Hamer HM, Morris HH, Mascha EJ, et al. Complications of invasive video-EEG monitoring with subdural grid electrodes. Neurology 2002;58(1):97–103.

81. Onal C, Otsubo H, Araki T, et al. Complications of invasive subdural grid monitoring in children with epilepsy. J Neurosurg 2003;98(5):1017–26.

82. Gonzalez Martinez F, Navarro Gutierrez S, de Leon Belmar JJ, et al. Electrocardiographic disorders associated to recent onset epilepsy. Neurologia 2005;20(10):698–701 [in Spanish].

83. Ozlen F, Asan Z, Tanriverdi T, et al. Surgical morbidity of invasive monitoring in epilepsy surgery: an experience from a single institution. Turkish Neurosurg 2010;20(3):364–72.

84. Afif A, Chabardes S, Minotti L, et al. Safety and usefulness of insular depth electrodes implanted via an oblique approach in patients with epilepsy. Neurosurgery 2008;62(5 Suppl 2):ONS471–9 [discussion: 479–80].

85. Nobili L, Cardinale F, Magliola U, et al. Taylor's focal cortical dysplasia increases the risk of sleep-related epilepsy. Epilepsia 2009;50(12):2599–604.

86. Serletis D, Bulacio J, Alexopoulos A, et al. Tailored unilobar and multilobar resections for orbitofrontal-plus epilepsy. Neurosurgery 2014;75(4):388–97 [discussion: 397].

Stereo-Encephalography Versus Subdural Electrodes for Seizure Localization

Irina Podkorytova, MD, Kathryn Hoes, MD, MBS,
Bradley Lega, MD*

KEYWORDS

- Stereo-encephalography (SEEG) • Subdural grids (SDG) or subdural electrodes (SDE)
- Epilepsy surgery

KEY POINTS

- Subdural electrode grids are traditionally used in North American epilepsy centers for intracranial seizure localization; improvements in technology have led to the popularization of stereo-encephalography (SEEG) using depth electrodes.
- Epilepsy surgery centers highest in volume now offer both subdural electrode and SEEG as intracranial strategies for seizure localization.
- The choice of technique is complex; it depends on the experience of the epilepsy surgical team as well as intrinsic patient characteristics.

INTRODUCTION

The stereo-encephalography (SEEG) method was developed in France by Jean Talairach and Jean Bancaud during the 1950s and has been mostly used in France and Italy as the method of choice for invasive localization in refractory focal epilepsy.[1] Its application in the United States has not been widely adopted until the past 5 years. Subdural grids and strips are the most common method for seizure localization used in North America. Large-volume epilepsy surgery centers now offer both subdural electrode (SDE) and SEEG for seizure localization. The choice of technique can be complex, and will depend on the experience and comfort of the epilepsy surgical team as well as patient characteristics. We offer in this article a general guide for considering SEEG along with SDE. These general guidelines have a footing in our experience with both techniques. **Table 1** describes some advantages and disadvantages of each strategy. **Table 2** describes several paradigmatic epilepsy types and how well SDE and SEEG apply to each. This table illustrates how candidates for SEEG or SDE surgical approach are selected at our institution.

The first principle we use in choosing an implantation strategy is to determine whether or not a lesion is present, and if this lesion is thought to correlate with the ictal onset area. If such a lesion is located adjacent to eloquent motor, visual, or speech cortex, we generally favor a grid electrode investigation, perhaps augmented with selected depth electrodes. If seizure semiology includes dyscognitive features that imply early involvement or primary onset in hippocampal-cingulate-insular areas, even with an associated lesion, we mostly prefer to start with stereo-electroencephalogram investigations.

Department of Neurological Surgery, University of Texas Southwestern Medical Center, 6363 Forest park road, Dallas, TX 75235, USA
* Corresponding author. 5323 Harry Hines Boulevard, Dallas, TX 75390-8548, USA
E-mail address: bradley.lega@utsouthwestern.edu

Neurosurg Clin N Am 27 (2016) 97–109
http://dx.doi.org/10.1016/j.nec.2015.08.008
1042-3680/16/$ – see front matter © 2016 Elsevier Inc. All rights reserved.

Table 1
A schematic for understanding technique advantages, limitations, and the best surgical candidates for both SDE and SEEG

	SDE	SEEG
Advantages	Accurate anatomic electrical/functional mapping of covered brain surfaces. Monitoring and resection within one hospital stay.	Enhanced targeting capability for deeper targets. Improved bihemispheric monitoring as well as mapping of functional networks. More facile placement in the reoperated patient. Given smaller access to implant leads, lessened wound healing morbidity.
Limitations	Difficulty in coverage of intrasulcal, deep brain and interhemispheric targets. Multilobar or bilateral sampling challenges. Morbidity associated with surgery: infectious consequences, hemorrhage, cerebral edema, if following previous surgery potential for adhesions and difficult dissection. Inaccuracy encountered when SDG used with additional depth electrodes.	Functional mapping restricted. If hemorrhage associated with placement of leads, can be large scale with significant consequences.
Ideal surgical candidates	The patient with a possible cortical target/lesion within eloquent cortex, a virgin surgical resection and/or goal of surgery to perform cortical mapping.	The patient with nonlesional MRI, deep lesions or EZ; and/or the previously operated patient. Also, the patient in whom bilateral exploration is required.

Abbreviations: EZ, epileptic zone; SDE, subdural electrode; SEEG, stereo-encephalography.

A second guiding principle is concern for bilaterality. For suspected frontal or fronto-parietal onset locations in which we believe bilateral sampling is important, we favor stereo EEG. If onset is clearly unilateral, either stereo EEG or grid recordings can be used. At our institution, if we believe good para-falcine sampling is important, we prefer stereo EEG, although other centers use multiple custom-designed grids or strips. For bilateral temporal lobe sampling, stereo EEG is preferable to burr hole strip electrocorticography (EcoG) investigations, we believe. Posttraumatic epilepsy often falls into this category, although individual examples may differ. Recording effectively from the insula requires stereo EEG.

A third simple principle we adopt is to use stereo EEG in patients who have undergone a previous craniotomy. The morbidity of placing subdural grids in a scarred subarachnoid space, wound and cerebrospinal fluid (CSF) leak issues after grid placement, and the limitations of the previous incision all lead us to prefer stereo EEG in this situation. Grid electrodes after a previous craniotomy would be for unusual circumstances.

Table 2
The favored epilepsy types for SEEG versus SDE techniques

SEEG	SEEG or SDE	SDE
Suspected bitemporal onset Insular onset Nodular heterotopia or tuberous sclerosis with multiple lesions Post craniotomy	Temporal/temporal plus (unilateral) SMA/Midline Occipital Lesion negative near motor cortex	Cortical lesion, near motor cortex Onset is suspected near the language cortex

Note the overlap with between the two techniques.
Abbreviations: SDE, subdural electrode; SEEG, stereo-encephalography; SMA, supplementary motor area.

Other, more specific patient situations are described later in this article. Different details of semiology and surface EEG patterns in suspected temporal lobe epilepsy present the richest variety and most nuanced decision making, which we attempt to recapitulate through a series of case examples.

BRIEF DESCRIPTION OF OUR INSTITUTIONAL STEREO-ENCEPHALOGRAPHY METHODOLOGY AND PROTOCOL

SEEG electrode implantation is planned according to a hypothesis for localized seizure onset combining surface EEG with careful review of seizure semiology and radiographic findings. In our practice with SEEG, electrode trajectories are calculated using neuronavigation software with calculations rendered for frame-based or frameless stereotaxy. Preoperative magnetic resonance or computed tomography (CT) angiography is performed to ensure the absence of vascular structures along the anticipated electrode trajectory. Electrode implantation is performed under general anesthesia. A robotic assistant device (such as the robotic system ROSA; Medtech, Montpellier, France) facilitates increased accuracy and reduced operative time, although frame-based or frameless strategies are also used. Electrodes traverse the skull through small twist-drill access sites and are fixed in place for the duration of recording by bolts seated within the bone of the cranial vault (**Fig. 1**). Electrodes may be inserted using orthogonal or oblique orientation. Intraoperatively, fluoroscopy is obtained to confirm the general accuracy of implanted electrode trajectories in real time. A postimplantation volumetric CT of the brain without contrast is obtained from the post anesthesia care unit. From the CT data set fused with the preoperative MRI, final verification of electrode placement is achieved. With assurance of targeting fidelity, initiation of recording in the monitored epilepsy ward commences. At the completion of recording, SEEG electrodes are removed in the operating room under local anesthesia with sedation as needed. Based on the intracranial SEEG recording, resective surgery is scheduled 2 to 3 months following SEEG electrode removal. This article is organized according to different seizure-onset hypotheses and explains our reasoning for choosing one approach or another.

STEREO-ENCEPHALOGRAPHY AS THE PREFERRED METHOD OF INVASIVE EVALUATION
Bitemporal Lobe Epilepsy

We perform bilateral SEEG explorations for MRI lesion-negative cases with bilateral interictal

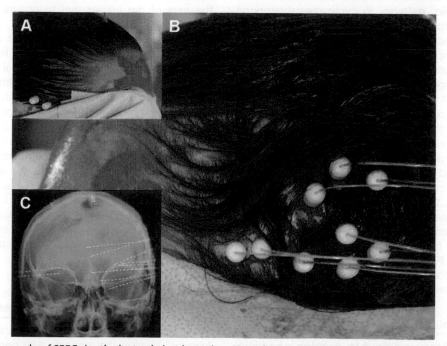

Fig. 1. An example of SEEG depth electrode implantation. Here the targets are the right temporal operculum and the insula (*A*), left perisylvian region, including frontal, temporal, and parietal operculum and insula, and lateral, inferior, and mesial temporal structures (*B*). A corresponding, intraoperative anteroposterior skull radiograph demonstrating bilateral implantation of SEEG electrodes (*C*). Note: Implantation is possible without hair shaving.

activity, variable surface EEG patterns, or with semiology that does not match the surface EEG pattern observed. In cases with bilateral radiographic changes, such as bilateral mesial temporal sclerosis, we use SEEG to confirm the laterality of seizures and to help guide placement of Neuropace (Mountain View, California, USA) electrodes or other palliative options if resection cannot be contemplated.

Signs of mesial temporal sclerosis on MRI do not exclude the possibility of neocortical temporal onset, extratemporal, or dual pathology (discussed later in this article). For instance, seizure onset from the temporal lobe opposite to subdural grid (SDG) placement is a known etiology of SDG-guided resection failure.[2] Seizures from the nondominant mesial temporal lobe may be clinically silent or not recognized by the patient or care providers. We feel standard practice should be to place at least one electrode into each hippocampus, or hippocampus and entorhinal/perirhinal/anterior fusiform cortex in lesion-negative cases without obvious semiological lateralization. However, other combinations of contralateral SEEG placement have been described, such as the hippocampus and insula or hippocampus and frontal operculum. This position is supported by data from implanted Neuropace devices. These data, in some patients, confirms that mesial temporal lobe seizures may have "cyclic" patterns. In cyclic mesial temporal seizures, epileptiform discharges are seen during a prolonged period of time (up to several months) in one temporal lobe but may periodically be recorded from the opposite temporal lobe during the next prolonged period of time.[3] Hence, we prefer bilateral temporal lobe sampling in most cases of suspected temporal lobe seizure onset.

In brief, the typical temporal SEEG exploration should include all temporal lobe cortices covering the hemisphere of the most probable seizure origin,[4] and at least one electrode always should be placed into the opposite mesial temporal structures (**Fig. 2**). If a patient's clinical data strongly imply bilateral temporal seizure onset, mirror limbic system exploration should be performed bilaterally (broad symmetric bilateral temporal coverage; **Fig. 3**). Bilateral coverage by one electrode is possible for anterior cingulate and orbitofrontal areas (**Fig. 4**).

Insular Epilepsy

Insular epilepsy is difficult to diagnose in pediatric and adult populations based on clinical semiology alone. It may mimic other seizure types (except occipital originating syndromes). Isnard and colleagues[5] described 6 patients with SEEG-recorded insular seizures that occurred in full consciousness, beginning with a sensation of laryngeal constriction and paresthesia, often unpleasant, affecting large cutaneous territories. It was eventually followed by dysarthric speech and focal motor convulsive symptoms. Dylgeri and colleagues[6] described 10 pediatric patients with SEEG-recorded insular seizures in which semiology varied from complex partial to hypermotor to purely autonomic semiology. Vadera and colleagues[2(p726)] reported 14 patients who underwent SEEG evaluation after previous SDE placement failure. Four (35%) of these 14 patients had insular (1) or fronto-insular (3) SEEG seizure onset on SEEG recording.

Given the anatomy of the Sylvian fissure with intertwined vasculature, SDE intracranial recording is not feasible without extensive surgical dissection and high risk of morbidity. Hence, SEEG is a preferable method when an insular onset is suspected, as it can circumvent this difficulty at the time of placement. We use an implantation array that covers temporal, frontotemporal, temporoparietal, frontotemporoparietal, and temporoparietooccipital trajectories that may be unilateral or bilateral, according to preimplantation hypothesis. Insular electrodes may be inserted using orthogonal or oblique orientation (**Fig. 5**), but we prefer at least one electrode that is aimed precisely along the axis of the insular gyri to ensure adequate sampling.

Temporal electrodes and opercular electrodes at their depth can be used to sample from the insula as well. We aim to have bilateral sampling, ideally bilateral insular coverage, although this may differ on a case-by-case basis. In our experience, the morbidity of insular sampling due to arterial injury is quite low. Instances of postoperative hemorrhage near the operculum we have encountered have been venous and cortically based. It is thought that the turgor and elastic properties of the middle cerebral arterial tree allow the vessels to be displaced by passing electrodes readily as compared with smaller cortical veins or arteries. Experience and caution with surgical trajectory planning are an obvious necessity.

Periventricular Nodular Heterotopia and Tuberous Sclerosis with Multiple Lesions

Tassi and colleagues[7] and Aghakhini and colleagues[8] posited that patients with periventricular nodular heterotopia warrant exploration of neocortex, mesial temporal structures, and heterotopic nodules. SEEG offers the benefit of sampling

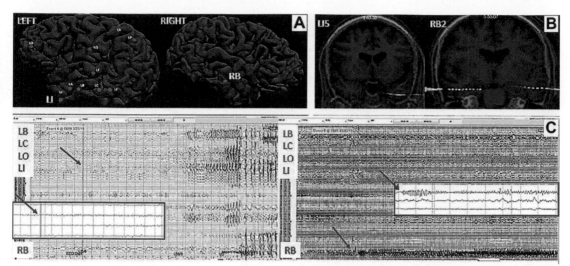

Fig. 2. Patient with weekly auras of déjà vu feeling followed by blank staring; scalp EEG showed left anterior temporal seizures and interictal sharp waves. (*A*) Typical left temporal stereoelectrode coverage with one right-sided electrode placed into the right anterior hippocampus. (*B*) Left: LI5 contact (*red dot*): left perirhinal cortex, where the onset of most seizures was recorded. Right: RB2 contact (*red dot*): right anterior hippocampus. There was a recorded clinical seizure from the right RB mesial contacts with an aura of "warm sensation," which was never reported as a seizure previously. (*C*) Left tracing: SEEG onset at the LI electrode mesial contacts (*red arrow*); zoomed window: LI5 contact (left perirhinal cortex). Right tracing: SEEG seizures started from the right anterior hippocampus (*red arrow*); zoomed window: RB2 contact onset. A Neuropace is implanted after this SEEG evaluation, and 2 seizures are captured at the time of report; the first seizure arose from the left mesial temporal structures, and the second seizure showed the right mesial temporal onset.

from multiple subcortical locations to identify which of several possible radiographic lesions is associated with seizure onset. As such, SEEG also may have an important role in selected cases of tuberous sclerosis, when there is clinical and EEG evidence of localized ictal onset in spite of bilateral or multifocal tubers.[9,10]

Fig. 6 demonstrates a patient with multiple tubers, including the left perirolandic area. The patient underwent SEEG at our institution and subsequently epileptogenic focus resection. This patient's seizures were localized to the posterior paracentral lobule, and we performed an awake craniotomy to maximize safe resection. In this case, surface EEG and semiology did not clearly correlate with a single lesion. Our concern was for onset in the supplementary motor area (SMA) region (due to negative motor ictal phenomenon) versus a perirolandic onset. If this patient did not have tuberous sclerosis, with multiple potential causative lesions, we believe that interhemispheric grid electrode exploration would also have been a reasonable option. However, sampling from the depths of sulci here and from the midcingulate region would have been notably limited. Moreover, this case illustrates the utility of SEEG for bilateral frontal lobe sampling, which we believe is necessary in most lesion-negative (or multilesion) cases with concern for frontal lobe onset.

Previous Craniotomy

Technical challenges associated with SDG implantation following previous craniotomy are mainly due to cortical adhesions.[11] Repeat craniotomy for SDE may be associated with additional scar formation as well as inability to assess to deeper structures. SEEG circumvents the dissection requisite for SDG implantation. SEEG has demonstrated accuracy in patients who have undergone previous craniotomy even in the presence of significant structural derangements, such as lobectomies or encephalomalacia. In a recent SEEG series, the accuracy of SEEG evaluation (along with magnetoencephalography) in patients who had previous craniotomy was studied in 29 patients; 21 of them achieved Engel I epilepsy surgery outcome after SEEG-guided resection.[12] Complications rate is low per a study from a large center that reported 14 patients who underwent SEEG implantation after SDE placement failure, and only 1 patient had major complication (brain abscess).[2(p725)] See **Fig. 7** for an illustrative case.

SUBDURAL ELECTRODES AS THE PREFERRED METHOD OF INVASIVE EVALUATION
Onset Near Language Cortex

We believe SDG placement is the preferred method of evaluation if the hypothesis is that

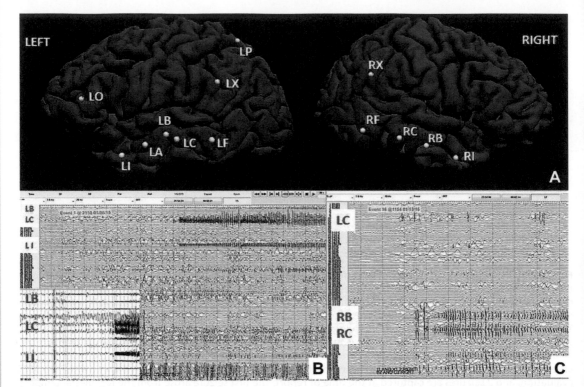

Fig. 3. The SEEG from this patient recorded seizures arising from the left and right hippocampus. In (*A*), typical bitemporal SEEG coverage is demonstrated. Leads demonstrated in the left 3-dimensional reconstruction are left side (from anterior to posterior): LO, orbitofrontal (bilateral coverage with one electrode); LI, temporal pole; LA, amygdala; LB, anterior hippocampus; LC, posterior hippocampus; LF, posterior temporal; LX, posterior cingulate; LP, precuneus. Also in (*A*), the leads demonstrated in the right 3-dimensional reconstruction are the right (from anterior to posterior): RI, temporal pole; RB, anterior hippocampus; RC, posterior hippocampus; RX, posterior cingulate; RF, posterior temporal. (*B*) SEEG seizure onset from the left anterior hippocampus (LB1 maximum); bipolar montage, 30-second page. Left lower corner: magnified picture of seizure onset; bipolar montage; fragment of 60-second page. (*C*) SEEG seizure onset started from the right anterior hippocampus (RB2 maximum).

seizure onset is located near Wernicke or Broca areas. This is especially true if a lesion is identified within these locations. Evaluation of perisylvian epilepsy includes language mapping. SDG with inclusion of depth electrodes may be the method of choice if seizure onset is suspected in the posterosuperior temporal gyrus (including the auditory cortex), temporoparietal junction, or frontal operculum of the dominant hemisphere. Suspicion of seizure onset near the language cortex could be

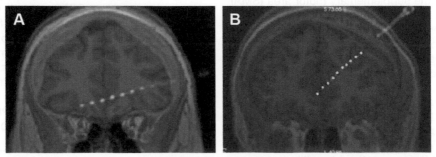

Fig. 4. Bilateral coverage by one electrode. (*A*) Orbitofrontal, oblique electrode orientation. (*B*) Anterior cingulate, oblique electrode orientation.

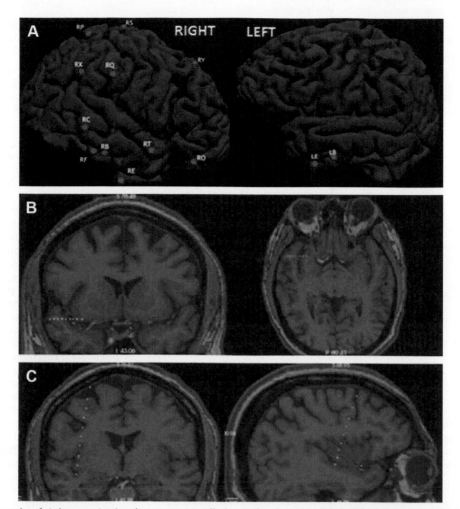

Fig. 5. Example of right anterior insular coverage. All electrodes shown in (A). In (B), the RT electrode is shown in an orthogonal right anterior insula electrode insertion, coronal and axial views. In (C), the RY electrode is shown in an oblique right posterior insula electrode insertion, coronal and sagittal views.

due to the semiology, such as peri-ictal aphasia, including aura. Combinations of SEEG electrodes with a small sampling of subdural strips (placed via a burr hole)[13] also have been described and may be useful in such situations.

Cortical Lesions: Gangliomas, Cavernomas, or Focal Cortical Dysplasia

When the lesion is well-circumscribed, such as in gangliomas or cavernomas, we recommend SDE to identify a precise margin to the onset zone. For focal cortical dysplasia, especially outside the temporal lobe, either SEEG or SDE can be used to pinpoint the ictal onset localization. Cortical dysplasia in the temporal pole, which can be radiographically occult or difficult to diagnose, is a classic example of such a phenomenon. For dysplasia, even an identifiable lesion can be misleading, because the ictal onset area may be somewhat removed from the radiographic abnormality, especially for type II dysplasia.[14–16]

LESIONS WHEREBY SUBDURAL ELECTRODE AND STEREO-ENCEPHALOGRAPHY YIELD COMPARABLE OUTCOMES
Temporal Plus Epilepsy

In temporal plus epilepsy (TPE), patients suffer from a more complex epileptogenic network that can encompass the temporal lobe as well as regions of the brain to which it is closely related, such as the orbitofrontal cortex, the insula, the frontal and parietal opercula, and the temporoparietooccipital junction. Based on seizure semiology only, it is difficult to distinguish among these syndromes. It is well recognized that some cases of extratemporal epilepsy syndromes can be mistaken for temporal lobe epilepsy on the basis of both semiology and surface EEG.[17] Insular,[18–20]

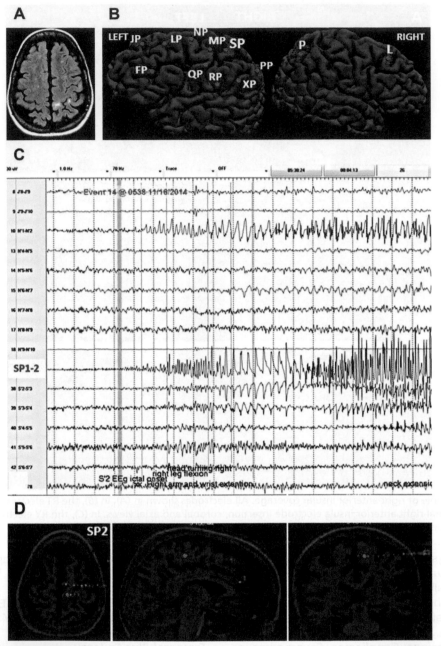

Fig. 6. A case of a patient with tuberous sclerosis. The described seizures were of somatosensory aura of right leg numbness or tingling leading to leg paralysis. Ictal scalp EEG was nonlocalizing. Following SEEG evaluation, left parietal awake craniotomy for resection of the epileptogenic focus with ECoG was performed; the patient has expected right foot numbness following surgery, no motor deficit (surgery recently completed). (*A*) Fluid-attenuated inversion recovery sequence on MRI showing a left superior parietal lobule tuber. (*B*) SEEG coverage breakdown. Left side: JP, superior frontal gyrus; FP, fronto-limbic anterior/inferior frontal gyrus; LP, superior frontal gyrus/middle frontal gyrus; NP, anterior cingulate/middle frontal gyrus; MP, paracentral lobule/middle frontal gyrus; QP, middle cingulate/precentral gyrus; RP, periopercular/inferior frontal gyrus; SP, paracentral lobule/precentral gyrus/postcentral gyrus; XP, posterior cingulate/supramarginal gyrus; PP, posterior cingulate/ superior parietal lobule/supramarginal gyrus. Right side: L, superior frontal gyrus/middle frontal gyrus; P, posterior cingulate/superior parietal lobule/supramarginal gyrus. SP: the electrode where seizure onset was observed. (*C*) SEEG seizure onset on SP2 contact (*green line*): paracentral lobule mesial, posterior to primary motor cortex, consistent with localization of left superior parietal lobule tuber. Bipolar montage, 30-second page. (*D*) SP2 contact localization, axial, sagittal, and coronal views.

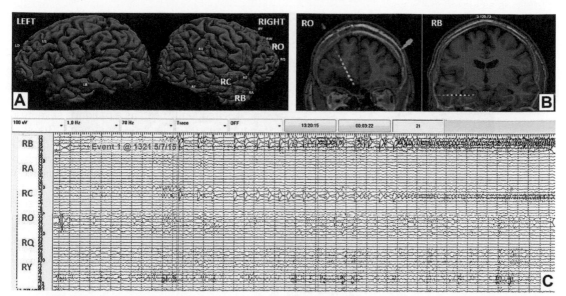

Fig. 7. Here a patient had a traumatic brain injury with subsequent bicoronal craniotomy and anterior cranial fossa repair. Corresponding MRI of the brain showed right frontal encephalomalacia. Surface EEG showed right anterior temporal seizure onset and interictal sharp waves. All SEEG seizures were recorded from the right hippocampus. In (A), the patient's implantation array with standard temporal coverage on the right side and additional electrodes placed in the bilateral frontal areas of encephalomalacia. One electrode was placed into the left hippocampus. In (B), right image, the RO electrode is located in the right frontal postcraniotomy area of encephalomalacia. In (B), left image, the RB electrode is located in the right anterior hippocampus. In (C), the tracing demonstrates electrographic seizures with onset in the anterior hippocampus (RB mesial contacts), spreading to the posterior hippocampus only (RC mesial contacts); no correlating clinical signs were observed during this seizures. RO (right orbito-frontal, encephalomalacia area), RQ (right anterior cingulate), and RY (right insula) electrodes presented in this tracing do not show seizure activity.

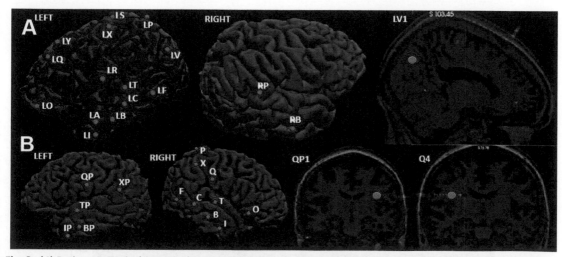

Fig. 8. (A) Patient A: Typical temporal coverage on the left side with electrodes placed into hippocampus (RB) and insula (RP) on the right side. The LV electrode placed into the primary visual cortex on the left side due to presence of visual auras. LS electrode covers area of encephalomalacia seen on MRI. SEEG seizure onset: left mesial temporal. (B) Patient B: Typical temporal coverage on the right side with electrodes placed into the temporal pole (IP), hippocampus (BP), insula (TP), and posterior cingulate (XP) on the left side. QP and Q electrodes are placed into the left and right parietal operculum, respectively, due to presence of somatosensory aura of tongue numbness. SEEG seizure onset: right mesial temporal.

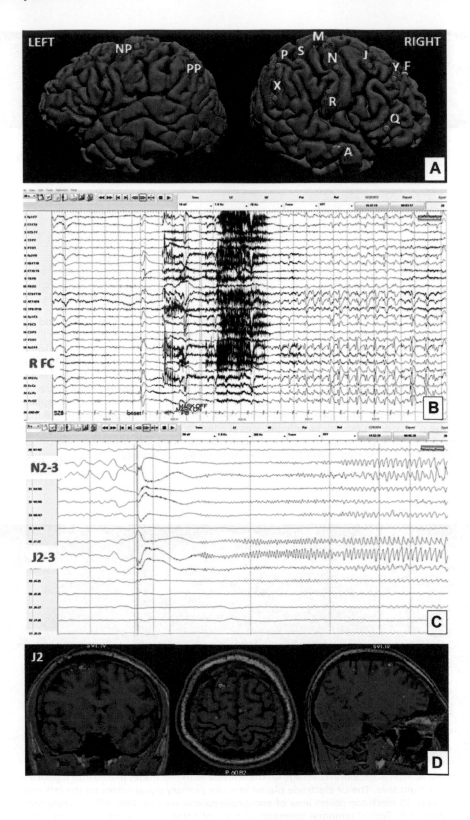

orbitofrontal (most frequent),[21] and cingulate gyrus[22] epilepsy can mimic the clinical features of temporal lobe epilepsy. Also, some seizures arising in extratemporal areas can remain nearly asymptomatic until they spread to the temporal lobe, where the temporal lobe epilepsy syndrome is triggered and recorded (eg, occipital[23] and parietal[24] epilepsy).

TPE should be considered if patients have sensory auras and for such cases we recommend exploration of sensory cortices together with traditional temporal implantation, as shown in **Fig. 8**. The choice of SEEG versus grid electrodes for these seizure types requires tradeoffs between the two approaches. SEEG offers the chance to cover areas that can mimic temporal lobe semiology, as described previously, which is difficult with SDEs. SEEG also provides highly accurate differential sampling from mesial structures, such as entorhinal cortex, amygdala, and both anterior and posterior hippocampus (see **Figs. 2** and **3**). However, if a surgeon seeks to limit the cortical resection without removing the entire temporal lobe, SDE can potentially identify a smaller ictal-onset location. Also, SDEs provide better anterior-posterior demarcation of the ictal onset if seizures start from an area outside the standard approximately 5-cm resection margin for temporal lobectomies.

Supplementary Motor Area/Midline Frontal or Parietal

When SMA onset is suspected, or for midline parietal onset, as in leg sensory semiology, accurate SDG placement can be an intraoperative challenge given venous anatomy. Additionally, deep midline structures, such as the cingulate gyrus, are hard to target with SDG. It is of note that when ictus is within the SMA, seizures tend to spread within this area before spreading to other regions. As such, 4 to 5 SEEG electrodes would be sufficient to sample the SMA, with a single electrode placed within the motor cortex to prove onset is not from the rolandic cortex (**Fig. 9**).

Mapping techniques, such as functional MRI and intraoperative cortical mapping, can be performed to localize the motor and sensory cortices. Accurately placed SEEG electrodes can serve to confirm anatomic location but not as well for defining a safe resection for eloquent areas. It follows that SDG more clearly demonstrates margins of eloquent motor function if there are significant anatomic derangements or if the onset location is actually within the motor or sensory cortex. We generally use SEEG for cases with suspected parafalcine onset (including SMA) because of concern for rapid bilateral spread and difficulty in obtaining bilateral parafalcine sampling with SDE.

Occipital Onset

Based on semiology and surface EEG with suspected occipital onset, if a lesion is present, we generally favor SDE placed to surround the lesion so that if surgical resection were to proceed, the maximal sparing of visual function could be achieved. In the absence of a lesion with suspected occipital onset, we prefer SEEG. This is preferred given the ability to sample deep sulcal structures, such as the calcarine fissure. In cases in which we are considering a large occipital resection with associated visual field loss, we prefer SEEG.

Onset Near the Motor Cortex

With lesions near the primary motor cortex, SDEs offer the advantage of precise mapping of the

Fig. 9. A representative case of a patient with nonlesional MRI and frequent auras and rare secondary generalized tonic clonic. Hypothesis: right mesial frontal onset was suspected, so right frontal SEEG coverage was performed; 1 electrode was placed to amygdala due to presence of fear aura, and 2 electrodes covering left SMA and left mesial parietal area were inserted to capture possible left mesial frontocentral ictal onset. (*A*) Implantation array right side (anterior to posterior): F, superior frontal gyrus; Q, anterior cingulate/inferior frontal gyrus; Y, posterior insula/middle frontal gyrus (oblique); J, superior frontal gyrus/middle frontal gyrus; A, amygdala/middle temporal gyrus; R, midcingulate/middle frontal gyrus; N, SMA anterior/middle frontal gyrus; M, SMA posterior/middle frontal gyrus (oblique); S, paracentral lobule/superior parietal lobule; X, posterior cingulate/supramarginal gyrus; P, precuneus/superior parietal lobule. Implantation array left side: NP, SMA/middle frontal gyrus; PP, precuneus/superior parietal lobule. (*B*) Scalp EEG showed right frontocentral seizure onset, R FC: right frontocentral electrode. (*C*) SEEG seizure onset on J2 contact within the superior frontal gyrus with fast spread to the N mesial contacts (SMA anterior). Green line: EEG seizure onset, pink line: clinical seizure onset (aura of "shaky" feeling). Of note, extraoperative stimulation of J1-2 contacts revealed "shaky" sensation, mouth numbness, and slowness of verbal response; J2-3: "eyes numbness" and slowness of verbal response; N1-2: head turn back and to the right; N 2 to 3: eyes and head version to the left, left leg jerking. Resection of seizure focus in the right superior frontal gyrus and right SMA was performed using cortex mapping with ECoG and electrical stimulation. Patient is several months seizure free on antiepileptic drugs without motor deficit. (*D*) Views of the J2 electrode in coronal, axial and sagittal planes.

ictal-onset zone versus areas of normal functioning. This supports surgical decision making when resection is undertaken. However, when semiology suggests the possibility of a lesion-plus onset location (ie, prerolandic or postrolandic onset locations), then SEEG may be preferable to achieve a wider sampling area, including the cingulate gyrus and insula. Some centers prefer SEEG for these cases, as intraoperative cortical mapping is a straightforward means of defining boundaries to a resection corridor. In our experience, we find case-by-case decision making for onset near motor cortex especially pertinent. For instance, if the preoperative hypothesis suggests an anatomically wide range of locations or a need for bilateral sampling, as in rapid spread from one lobe to another, we find SEEG may be advisable. See **Fig. 6** for an illustrative case.

SUMMARY

The approaches for invasive evaluation of "difficult-to-localize" epilepsies are debated between epilepsy treatment centers. The treatment paradigm for each patient is always individualized in our practice. From our experience, we have found a set of paradigmatic cases that are better candidates for SEEG or SDE. For cases in which both approaches offer advantages, we select an electrode implantation method based on individual patient characteristics. Each center will likely arrive at its own "point of equilibrium" between SEEG and SDE. We offer our experience as a guide to help surgical epilepsy teams in making this decision.

REFERENCES

1. Bancaud J, Angelergues R, Bernouilli C, et al. Functional stereotactic exploration (SEEG) of epilepsy. Electroencephalogr Clin Neurophysiol 1970;28(1): 85–6.
2. Vadera S, Mullin J, Bulacio J, et al. Stereoelectroencephalography following subdural grid placement for difficult to localize epilepsy. Neurosurgery 2013; 72(5):723–9.
3. Smart O, Rolston JD, Epstein DM, et al. Hippocampal seizure-onset laterality can change over long timescales: a same-patient observation over 500 days. Epilepsy Behav Case Rep 2013;1:56–61.
4. Gonzalez-Martinez J, Mullin J, Bulacio J, et al. Stereoelectroencephalography in children and adolescents with difficult-to-localize refractory focal epilepsy. Neurosurgery 2014;75(3):258–68.
5. Isnard J, Guenot M, Sindou M, et al. Clinical manifestations of insular lobe seizures: a stereo-electroencephalographic study. Epilepsia 2004; 45(9):1079–90.
6. Dylgeri S, Taussig D, Chipaux M, et al. Insular and insulo-opercular epilepsy in childhood: an SEEG study. Seizure 2014;23(4):300–8.
7. Tassi L, Colombo N, Cossu M, et al. Electroclinical, MRI and neuropathological study of 10 patients with nodular heterotopia, with surgical outcomes. Brain 2005;128(pt 2):321–37.
8. Aghakhani Y, Kinay D, Gotman J, et al. The role of periventricular nodular heterotopia in epileptogenesis. Brain 2005;128(pt 3):641–51.
9. Akalan N, Di Rocco C. Pediatric epilepsy surgery. Acta Neurochirurgica 2014;156(10):2023.
10. Novengo F, Massimi L, Di Rocco C. Epilepsy in tuberous sclerosis complex. Adv Tech Stand Neurosurg 2012;39:131–63.
11. Gonzalez-Martinez J, Najm M. Indications and selection criteria for invasive monitoring in children with cortical dysplasia. Childs Nerv Syst 2014; 30(11):1823–9.
12. Podkorytova I, Murakami H, Wang I, et al. Use of MEG for re-evaluation of epilepsy patients after previous neurosurgery. American Epilepsy Society 68th Annual Meeting. Seattle (WA), December 7, 2014.
13. Enatsu R, Bulacio J, Najm I, et al. Combining stereo-electroencephalography and subdural electrodes in the diagnosis and treatment of medically intractable epilepsy. J Clin Neurosci 2014;21(8): 1441–5.
14. Widdess-Walsh P, Jeha L, Nair D, et al. Subdural electrode analysis in focal cortical dysplasia: predictors of surgical outcome. Neurology 2007;69(7): 660–7.
15. Marusic P, Najm I, Ying Z, et al. Focal cortical dysplasias in eloquent cortex: functional characteristics and correlation with MRI and histopathologic changes. Epilepsia 2002;43(1):27–32.
16. Ying Z, Najm I. Mechanisms of epileptogenicity in focal malformations caused by abnormal cortical development. Neurosurg Clin N Am 2002;13(1):27–33.
17. Lee KH, Park YD, King DW, et al. Prognostic implication of contralateral secondary electrographic seizures in temporal lobe epilepsy. Epilepsia 2000; 41(11):1444–9.
18. Isnard J, Guenot M, Ostrowsky K, et al. The role of the insular cortex in temporal lobe epilepsy. Ann Neurol 2000;48(4):614–23.
19. Ryvlin P. Beyond pharmacotherapy: surgical management. Epilepsia 2003;44(Suppl 5):23–8.
20. Harroud A, Bouthillier A, Weil AG, et al. Temporal lobe epilepsy surgery failures: a review. Epilepsy Res Treat 2012;2012:201651.
21. Shihabuddin B, Abou-Khalil B, Delbeke D, et al. Orbitofrontal epilepsy masquerading as temporal lobe epilepsy—a case report. Seizure 2001;10(2):134–8.

22. Devinsky O, Morrell MJ, Vogt BA. Contributions of anterior cingulate cortex to behavior. Brain 1995;118(pt 1):279–306.
23. Palmini A, Andermann F, Dubeau F, et al. Occipito-temporal epilepsies: evaluation of selected patients requiring depth electrodes studies and rationale for surgical approaches. Epilepsia 1993;34(1):84–96.
24. Williamson PD, Boon PA, Thadani VM, et al. Parietal lobe epilepsy: diagnostic considerations and results of surgery. Ann Neurol 1992;31(2):193–201.

Responsive Direct Brain Stimulation for Epilepsy

Martha J. Morrell, MD[a,b,*], Casey Halpern, MD[c]

KEYWORDS

- Closed-loop • Responsive • Stimulation • Epilepsy • Intractable • Intracranial • Electrocorticogram
- Neurostimulator

KEY POINTS

- Closed-loop responsive stimulation of the seizure focus reduces the frequency of medically intractable partial onset seizures from 44% at 1 year to 60% to 66% over 3 to 6 years of treatment.
- Risks of responsive stimulation as provided by the first responsive neurostimulator (RNS System) are similar to other implanted medical devices, and the neurostimulator can be programmed so that therapeutic stimulation is not perceived.
- There are improvements in quality of life with responsive stimulation and no negative effects on mood or cognition, and some patients experience improvements in aspects of language and memory.
- Quantitative electrophysiological data combined with clinical seizure counts are used to establish optimal detection and stimulation settings for each patient.
- Chronic ambulatory electrocorticographic monitoring provides information regarding the location(s) of the seizure focus and may provide biomarkers to measure disease activity.

INTRODUCTION

Neurostimulation is an increasingly important treatment modality for disorders of the nervous system.[1–4] Most neurostimulation devices are open-loop; stimulation settings are preprogrammed and do not automatically respond to changes in electrophysiological signals or the patient's clinical symptoms. Open-loop stimulation is effective in several clinical applications, including Parkinson's disease,[5,6] essential tremor,[7] dystonia,[8] pain,[9] and more recently, epilepsy.[10,11] However, because many neurologic disorders are not static conditions, there is increasing interest in neurostimulation approaches that adapt to changes in clinical symptoms or quantitative biomarkers.

In contrast to open-loop stimulation devices, responsive (or closed-loop) neurostimulation devices modulate or adapt therapy in response to physiologic signals, in addition to clinically overt symptoms, and may be more efficient, effective, and better tolerated than open-loop stimulation.[12,13] Responsive stimulation approaches are being explored for Parkinson's disease. Investigational closed-loop stimulation for Parkinson's disease provides stimulation in the subthalamic nucleus in response to changes in beta amplitude, with reports of improvements in motor function, speech, gait, and balance.[13–18]

This review focuses on targeted cortical responsive stimulation, which has been approved by the US Food and Drug Administration (FDA) for the

Disclosures: Dr M.J. Morrell is an employee of and has equity ownership/stock options with NeuroPace Inc. Dr C. Halpern does not have any conflicts of interest that are relevant to the subject matter or materials discussed in this article.

[a] NeuroPace, Inc, 455 North Bernardo Avenue, Mountain View, CA 94043, USA; [b] Department of Neurology and Neurological Sciences, Stanford University, Stanford, CA, USA; [c] Department of Neurosurgery, Stanford University, 300 Pasteur Drive A301, MC 5325, Stanford, CA 94305, USA
* Corresponding author. 455 North Bernardo Avenue, Mountain View, CA 94043.
E-mail address: mmorrell@neuropace.com

adjunctive treatment of epilepsy with partial onset seizures.

NEUROSTIMULATION FOR EPILEPSY

Epilepsy comprises a group of neurologic conditions characterized by recurrent seizures. The partial epilepsies (also known as localization-related epilepsy) are the most common type of epilepsy in adults, and at least one-third cannot achieve seizure control with antiepileptic medications.[19] One option for these patients is to resect the seizure focus.[20,21] However, many patients with partial onset seizures are not candidates for a cortical resection because the chance of a substantial seizure reduction is too low or the risk of a neurologic morbidity is too high. Moreover, not all patients who undergo resective procedures achieve seizure freedom. Approximately 30% to 40% of patients who undergo temporal lobectomies, which is the most common and most successful type of resective surgery, continue to have disabling seizures at 1 year after surgery.[20–22]

Neurostimulation is an option for some patients with medically intractable partial seizures who have either failed or are not candidates for resective surgery. There are currently two FDA-approved neurostimulation therapies for adjunctive treatment of medically intractable partial-onset epilepsy: vagus nerve stimulation (VNS) and responsive cortical stimulation. A third neurostimulation modality, open-loop deep brain stimulation of the anterior thalamic nucleus, is not approved in the United States as of the date this is written, but is approved in other countries.[11]

The VNS Therapy System (Cyberonics, Houston, TX, USA)[23] provides open-loop scheduled stimulation to the vagus nerve using a pectorally implanted pulse generator and electrodes wrapped around the left vagus nerve. Stimulation is typically delivered for 30 seconds every 5 minutes. External application of a magnet over the pulse generator triggers additional stimulation.

Average seizure reductions in patients with intractable partial onset seizures during the blinded period of randomized controlled trials of the VNS Therapy System were 24% to 28%[24,25] and were 35% to 44% at 2 years in open-label prospective studies.[26] Side effects related to stimulation of the vagus and recurrent laryngeal nerve include voice alteration (50%), increased coughing (41%), pharyngitis (27%), dyspnea (18%), dyspepsia (12%), nausea (19%), and laryngismus (3.2%).[24,27] A recently FDA-approved VNS model (Aspire SR; Cyberonics, Inc) activates stimulation when the heart rate exceeds a prespecified threshold in order to provide additional treatment for seizures that are accompanied by tachycardia (Aspire SR, Cyberonics, Inc).[23] It is unclear at this time if this device will prove to be more efficacious or better tolerated than its open-loop precursor.

A reduction in seizures has been reported in several small and uncontrolled studies of open-loop continuous or scheduled neurostimulation as well as in one randomized controlled trial.[28] Stimulation targets have included the cerebellum,[29] caudate nucleus,[30–32] centromedian nucleus,[31,33,34] subthalamic nucleus,[35] and hippocampus.[36–38] In the only randomized controlled trial of open-loop stimulation,[10] 110 adults with medically intractable partial onset seizures were randomized to scheduled or sham stimulation in the anterior nuclei of the thalamus on a schedule of 1 minute on and 5 minutes off. Patients treated with stimulation had a significantly greater reduction in seizures compared with the sham stimulation patients with an overall adjusted percent difference of −17% (P<.039).[10] The stimulated group had significantly more adverse events related to depression, memory, and concentration, but there were not differences between the groups by neuropsychological testing. The seizure reduction at 1 year was −41% and reached 57% to 65% in years 3 through 5.[10,11]

Closed-Loop Responsive Direct Brain Stimulation

Closed-loop responsive direct brain stimulation represents a new treatment paradigm for epilepsy. Seizures and epileptiform activity are sporadic and relatively infrequent, making an episodic treatment approach such as responsive stimulation an attractive option. Clinical observations and small studies have shown that electrographic seizures induced by electrical stimulation during brain mapping can be shortened or even terminated by immediately delivering a brief burst of electrical stimulation at the site of the discharge.[39–41] Other small studies in persons being evaluated with intracranial electrodes for epilepsy surgery have indicated that automated stimulation to the seizure focus delivered by investigational external devices was well tolerated and seemed to suppress electrographic and perhaps clinical seizures.[42–44]

The Responsive Neurostimulator System

The first implantable closed-loop responsive direct brain neurostimulator was approved in the United States in late 2013 as an adjunctive therapy in adults with medically uncontrolled partial onset seizures localized to 1 or 2 epileptogenic foci.[45]

The RNS System technology builds on decades-long experience in cardiac rhythm management devices. A neurostimulator continuously senses and monitors electrical activity from the brain (electrocorticographic activity) through 1 or 2 leads placed at the seizure focus and provides responsive electrical stimulation to the seizure focus when abnormal electrocorticographic activity prespecified by the physician occurs. The physician tailors detection and responsive stimulation for each patient according to the patient's report of their clinical response as well as the quantitative electrographic data that the device provides.

Components of the RNS System are illustrated in **Fig. 1**. The cranially seated neurostimulator is connected to 1 or 2 depth or cortical strip leads that are surgically placed in the brain at 1 or 2 seizure foci (**Fig. 2**). Each lead contains 4 electrodes, each of which can be used for both sensing and stimulating. The physician programs detection and stimulation settings and retrieves and reviews data provided by the neurostimulator, such as battery measurements, lead impedances, programmed settings, time and date of detection and stimulations, and samples of electrocorticograms. Up to 6 minutes of electrocorticogram samples can be stored at any one time. In order to clear neurostimulator memory for additional electrocorticogram (ECoG) storage, the patient transfers data from the neurostimulator to a home-use remote monitor daily to weekly. Patient data acquired by the physician's programmer or the patient's remote monitor are then transmitted over the Internet to the Patient Data Management System (PDMS), where it is securely stored and available for physician review.

Which electrocorticogram samples are stored is customizable and may include times of day when the patient swipes a magnet over the neurostimulator to indicate a clinical seizure, spike and slow waves, rhythmic changes in frequency, or other electrocorticographic patterns that are typical of electrographic seizures in that patient. This quantitative data may be used by the physician as one means by which to assess the response to therapy (**Fig. 3**).

The neurostimulator delivers current-controlled, charge-balanced biphasic pulses through any or all of the 8 electrodes. The physician programs stimulation frequency (1–333 Hz), current (0.5–12 mA), pulse-width (40–1000 μs), and duration (10–5000 ms). The most common stimulation settings in the clinical trials were a current of 1.5 to 3 mA, a pulse width of 160 μs, a stimulation burst duration of 100 to 200 ms, and a pulse frequency between 100 and 200 Hz. Usually, patients had 600 to 2000 detections and stimulations a day. At a typical burst duration of 100 to 200 ms, this is a total of less than 5 minutes of stimulation a day.[46]

The stimulation pathway is selected by the physician. Any combination of the 8 electrodes can be used for stimulation, and the neurostimulator housing (case) can be incorporated into the pathway as an indifferent electrode. Once an initial detection and stimulation occur, the neurostimulator can provide an additional 4 stimulations if the detected activity does not resolve. Each of these stimulations contains 2 bursts that are

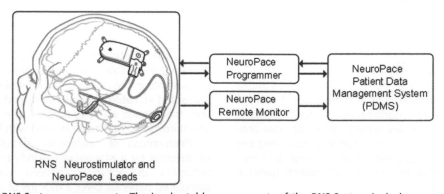

RNS Neurostimulator and
NeuroPace Leads

Fig. 1. The RNS System components. The implantable components of the RNS System include a neurostimulator and depth and cortical strip leads. Leads are selected based on the target. The programmer contains proprietary software and custom telemetry components to communicate with the neurostimulator. The programmer retrieves data stored on the neurostimulator and is used by the physician to program neurostimulator detection and stimulation settings. The remote monitor is a home-use monitoring device for the patient to retrieve data stored on the neurostimulator. The PDMS is a centralized database that contains data uploaded from the programmer and remote monitor. Neurostimulator data and detection settings can also be transferred from PDMS to the programmer. (© 2015 NeuroPace, Inc.)

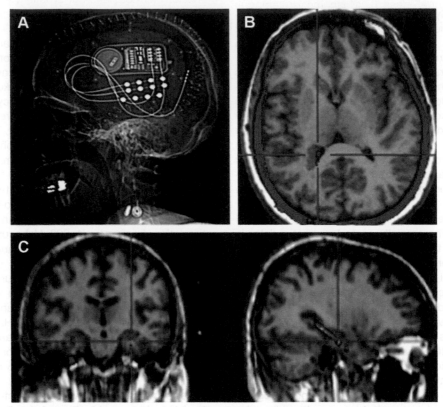

Fig. 2. RNS Neurostimulator and NeuroPace Lead implantation strategies. The neurostimulator is placed within the skull, generally in the parietal region. Depth leads and cortical strip leads are selected based on the seizure focus targets. (*A*) Four subcortical strip leads have been placed over lateral temporal cortex; 2 of these leads can be connected to the neurostimulator at any one time. (*B*) A depth lead is placed within a periventricular heterotopia. A second depth lead (not shown in this image) was placed longitudinally within in the right hippocampus. (*C*) A patient with bilateral mesial temporal lobe epilepsy has a longitudinally placed depth in the left and the right hippocampus. (© 2015 NeuroPace, Inc.)

individually programmed, providing the opportunity for several different types of stimulation within a given electrocorticographic discharge.

Clinical Experience

The RNS System is approved in the United States as an adjunctive therapy in individuals 18 years of age or older with partial onset seizures localized to 1 or 2 foci who are refractory to 2 or more antiepileptic medications and currently have frequent and disabling seizures (motor partial seizures, complex partial seizures, or secondarily generalized seizures).[45]

Safety and efficacy of the RNS System was established in 3 clinical trials: a 2-year primarily open-label safety study (Feasibility study, N = 65), a 2-year randomized controlled trial (Pivotal study, N = 191), and a 7-year long-term extension study (Long-term Treatment study, N = 230) for patients completing the Feasibility or Pivotal studies. In total, 256 patients were implanted within the RNS System trials.

The multicenter double-blinded randomized and sham-stimulation controlled Pivotal study demonstrated the safety and effectiveness of the RNS System for its indicated use. Demographics of the patients in the randomized controlled trial are presented in **Table 1**. Nearly one-third (32%) had prior therapeutic epilepsy surgery, and more than one-third (34%) had been treated with VNS.[1,47]

Effectiveness of responsive stimulation was established by a statistically significantly greater reduction in active compared with sham-stimulated patients. Over 3 months of the blinded period, the overall seizure reduction in the treated patients was 37.9% and 17.3% in the sham patients ($P = .012$).[47]

Seizure frequency month to month revealed a transient reduction in seizures of about 25% in the month after the implant procedure (before patients were randomized). Thereafter, the seizure

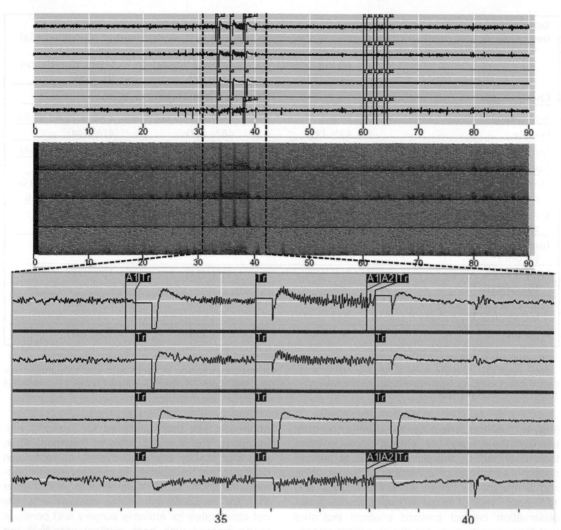

Fig. 3. The ECoG samples are reviewed on the programmer or the PDMS. Four channels of ECoG are displayed according to a bipolar montage using the 8 electrodes across 2 connected leads. The physician selects the electrocorticographic activity to be detected. One or more detection algorithms (bandpass, line-length, and area) are used by the neurostimulator to detect up to 4 specific patterns. Detection settings are then iteratively adjusted to optimize the sensitivity, specificity, and latency of the detection for that patient based on the physician's visual review of the electrocorticographic data. Data can be viewed as an electrocorticogram or as a frequency spectrum display. (A1, A2) Detections of specific prespecified patterns; Tr, a responsive stimulation. In this case, A1 has been programmed to detect low-frequency, low-amplitude activity on the first channel, and A2 has been programmed to detect similar activity on the fourth channel. The artifact seen after Tr represents the stimulation. (© 2015 NeuroPace, Inc.)

reduction continued to improve in the treated subjects, whereas the nontreated patients gradually approached their preimplant seizure frequency. By the final month of the blinded period (the fifth month after implant), patients treated with responsive stimulation had a reduction in seizures of 41.5% compared with a 9.4% seizure reduction in the sham-stimulated patients (generalized estimating equation [GEE] estimate, $P = .008$).[47]

Responsive stimulation was effective in patients with different clinical characteristics. A similar benefit was achieved in patients with mesial temporal lobe seizure onsets and with neocortical seizure onsets, when seizures arose from 1 or 2 foci, and with and without prior treatment with VNS. Patients who had already undergone a therapeutic epilepsy surgery were as likely to respond as those who had not.

All patients had the opportunity to receive responsive stimulation during the open-label period, and the seizure reduction continued to improve.[1] The median percent reduction in seizures was 44% at 1 year and 53% at 2 years and reached 60% to 66% at years 3 through 6

Table 1
Demographic and baseline characteristics of subjects in the RNS System randomized controlled trial

Characteristic	All Implanted (N = 191)	Active Stimulation (N = 97)	Sham Stimulation (N = 94)
	Mean ± SD (min-max) or % (n)		
Age (years)	34.9 ± 11.6 (18–66)	34.0 ± 11.5 (18–60)	35.9 ± 11.6 (18–66)
Female	48% (91)	48% (47)	47% (44)
Duration of epilepsy (years)	20.5 ± 11.6 (2–57)	20.0 ± 11.2 (2–57)	21.0 ± 12.2 (2–54)
Number of AEDs at enrollment	2.8 ± 1.2 (0–8)	2.8 ± 1.3 (1–8)	2.9 ± 1.1 (0–6)
Mean seizure frequency during preimplant period (seizures/mo)	34.2 ± 61.9 (3–338) median = 9.7	33.5 ± 56.8 (3–295) median = 8.7	34.9 ± 67.1 (3–338) median = 11.6
Seizure onset location–mesial temporal lobe only (vs other)[1]	50% (95)	49% (48)	50% (47)
Number of seizure foci–two (vs one)[a]	55% (106)	49% (48)	62% (58)
Prior therapeutic surgery for epilepsy[a]	32% (62)	35% (34)	30% (28)
Prior EEG monitoring with intracranial electrodes	59% (113)	65% (63)	53% (50)
Prior VNS	34% (64)	31% (30)	36% (34)

[a] Characteristics used as strata in randomization algorithm.
From Heck CN, King-Stephens D, Massey AD, et al. Two-year seizure reduction in adults with medically intractable partial onset epilepsy treated with responsive neurostimulation: final results of the RNS System Pivotal trial. Epilepsia 2014;55:435; with permission.

(Fig. 4).[1,2] Although no subject was entirely seizure free over the average 5.4 years of follow-up, more than one-third of the subjects had at least 1 seizure-free period of 3 months or longer, 23% had 6 months or longer without a seizure, and 13% had 1 year or longer without seizures. A last observation carried forward analysis indicated that these results were not due to patient discontinuations. The improvements in seizure control did not correlate with changes in antiepileptic medications.

Serious adverse events during treatment with the RNS System were no worse than with implantation of intracranial electrodes and epilepsy surgery, or with treatment of Parkinson's disease with deep brain stimulation. Stimulation was well tolerated; there was no difference in the frequency or type of serious adverse events between the treated and sham groups over the blinded period. Device-related serious adverse events over 2 years were soft tissue infection at the implant site (3.7% at 2 years), revised leads (3.7%), and lead damage (2.6%). Over 1389 patient-implant–years, the risk of infection remained stable at about 3.5% with each neurostimulator procedure.[1,2]

Quality of life (QOL) is a treatment outcome that incorporates the global effect of a treatment. At baseline, QOL was substantially lower for the participants in the RNS System randomized

controlled trial than expected for persons with epilepsy. After 1 and 2 years of treatment, QOL was significantly improved overall, as well as in domains that are specific to epilepsy and to cognitive function. QOL improvements were higher than for medically intractable patients who are not candidates for epilepsy surgery and continue to be treated with best medical care,[48,49] but were not as high as for patients with medically intractable partial seizures who achieve seizure freedom after an epilepsy surgery.[50]

Depression and cognitive deficits are common in persons with epilepsy and could be exacerbated by brain stimulation. Sixteen percent of the 191 participants in the randomized controlled trial of the RNS System met standardized criteria for moderately severe depression at baseline.[3] There was no increase in the rate of depression over the 2 years of treatment, and validated inventories of mood showed modest improvements.

Comprehensive neuropsychological assessments showed that there were no group deteriorations from baseline in any of the 14 neurocognitive domains at the end of the blinded period or after 1 and 2 years of treatment.[4] In fact, patients with seizures beginning in a neocortical focus, especially in the frontal lobe, had statistically significant improvements in verbal fluency, and patients with seizures of mesial temporal lobe onset have

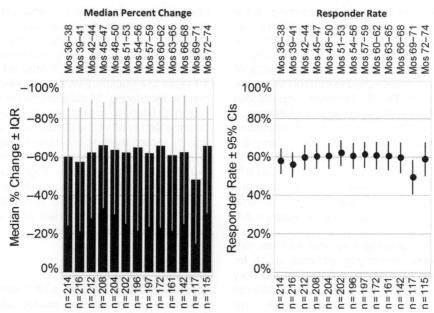

Fig. 4. Median percent seizure reduction (*left*) and responder rate (*rate*) from years 3 through 6 of the long-term treatment trial. The median percent change in total disabling seizures is plotted with the interquartile range (IQR) indicated by the error bars. Responder rates are plotted with error bars indicating the 95% confidence interval (CI; Wilson method). The response indicates that the effect of treatment with responsive neurostimulation is sustained over many years and suggests that patients do not habituate to the stimulation over time. The median percent change in seizures over the long term ranged from −48% (IQR: −15% to −86%) to −66% (IQR: −31% to −87%). Responder rates ranged from 56% (95% CI: 50% to 62%) to 62% (95% CI: 55% to 69%). (*From* Bergey GK, Morrell MJ, Mizrahi EM, et al. Long-term treatment with responsive brain stimulation in adults with refractory partial seizures. Neurology 2015;84:814; with permission.)

a modest but statistically significant improvement in learning, delayed free recall, and recognition. These results demonstrate that there is no overall risk to mood or cognition with treatment with responsive neurostimulation and that some patients may experience benefit.

Applications for Chronic Ambulatory Electrocorticographic Monitoring

Chronic ambulatory electrocorticographic data provide insight into the temporal dynamics of partial onset seizures that has not previously been available, and may supplement information obtained in the acute inpatient epilepsy monitoring unit. Clinical epileptologists have long been concerned that seizure frequency and semiology may change when patients are undergoing inpatient electroencephalography (EEG) monitoring.[51,52] In order to obtain seizures within an acceptable period of time in the inpatient setting (generally 1–2 weeks), a common practice is to rapidly reduce or withdraw antiepileptic medications and to perform other seizure-provoking maneuvers such as sleep deprivation. However, this short period of monitoring might be insufficient

to capture all of that patient's seizure onsets, and seizure-provoking strategies could elicit atypical electrographic activity and even atypical seizures.[53–56] An additional concern with intracranial EEG monitoring is that the electrophysiology could be acutely altered as a consequence of the electrode implantation.

Data from both trials of direct brain stimulation for partial epilepsy suggest these are valid concerns.[10,47] In both studies, there was an immediate reduction in seizure frequency after implantation of intracranial leads that was of similar magnitude and occurred before any patient received stimulation. Although patients treated with stimulation enjoyed progressive and significant improvements in seizure control, the nonstimulated patients had not completely returned to their preimplant baseline seizure frequency after several months. The mechanism of this implant effect is unknown but is unlikely to be related to a specific type of lesion because anatomic targets differed across the 2 studies (anterior nucleus of the thalamus and several areas within the cortex).

Another concern about acute electrocorticographic recordings is that these might not be representative of the chronic electrophysiology.[57–59]

Data obtained from patients participating in the RNS System randomized controlled trial[60] demonstrate that impedances for depth and subdural cortical electrodes are stable over the long term, providing confidence in the long-term quality of the electrographic data used to control responsive brain stimulation (**Fig. 5**). However, impedances did not stabilize for 4 months after implantation of depth leads and for 5 months after implantation of subdural leads. Although the mechanisms are not known, the time course suggests this may be related to microglial activation[61] or inflammation.[62] Whatever the cause of these postimplant changes in impedance, these observations raise concerns about the reliability of acute electrocorticographic recordings.

Limited time sampling may also limit the reliability of acute electrographic data used for seizure focus localization. Chronic ambulatory electrocorticography was reviewed in 82 patients in the RNS System randomized controlled trial who were implanted with bilateral mesial temporal lobe electrodes because the standard diagnostic evaluation (that included inpatient EEG monitoring as well as neuroimaging and functional assessments) had not conclusively established lateralization of the seizure focus.[63] After an average of 4.7 years of ambulatory intracranial electrocorticographic monitoring, 13 subjects had only unilateral seizures. Bilateral mesial temporal onsets were documented in 69 of the 82 subjects; the average time to record the first contralateral hippocampal seizure was 41.6 days (median 13 days, range 0–376 days) (**Fig. 6**). This average time suggests that chronic ambulatory monitoring may help to identify patients with mesial temporal lobe epilepsy who are likely to benefit from a resection as well as those who will not.

DISCUSSION

Controlled clinical trials in adults with medically intractable partial seizures treated with the RNS System demonstrate that closed-loop responsive

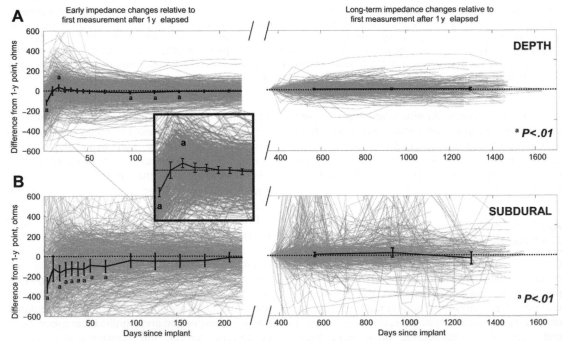

Fig. 5. Short-term impedance change (*left*) and long-term stability (*right*). Early changes (*left axes*) and long-term stability (*right axes*) in impedance are shown for electrodes on depth (*A*) and subdural leads (*B*). Each measurement for a given electrode is plotted relative to impedance at or nearest to the 1-year mark for that electrode. Modeled impedance change (*solid lines*), analogous to mean impedance change, and 99% CI (*vertical bars*) were determined by GEE modeling with weekly bins through day 56 and 4-week bins through day 224 (*left*), and yearly bins (*right*). Significant ([a] P<.01) early changes in depth leads (inset) include lower impedances from 2 to 4 months when compared with the 1-year mark. Early changes in subdural leads include lower impedance from weeks 1 through 12, with continued changes in impedance to 5 months. No significant long-term changes were observed after the 1-year mark. (*From* Sillay KA, Rutecki P, Cicora K, et al. Long-term measurement of impedance in chronically implanted depth and subdural electrodes during responsive neurostimulation in humans. Brain Stimul 2013;6(5):718–26; with permission.)

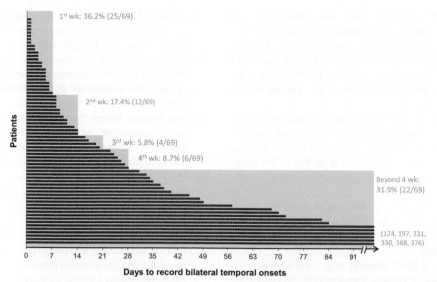

Fig. 6. Time to record bilateral temporal onsets. Randomizations occurred at 4 weeks postimplant (day 28). There was no difference between those randomized to responsive or sham stimulation in the time to record the first contralateral seizure (*P* = .51, two-sample *t* test). (*From* King-Stephens D, Mirro E, Weber PB, et al. Lateralization of mesial temporal lobe epilepsy with chronic ambulatory electrocorticography. Epilepsia 2015;56:964; with permission.)

neurostimulation to the seizure focus reduces the frequency of disabling seizures, is well tolerated, and is acceptably safe. Seizure reductions are evident with initiation of treatment and continue to increase over the longer term reaching median reductions of 60% to 66% with 3 to 6 years of treatment. Treatment with responsive cortical stimulation is also associated with improvements in QOL and cognitive functions related to the functional area being treated. Chronic ambulatory electrocorticographic monitoring provides quantitative data about interictal and ictal events as well as temporal patterns for seizures. The time and date–stamped records of all detection and stimulations and the electrocorticogram samples represent a rich data set that has not previously been available and contributes to the understanding of each patient's disease in ways that may enhance disease management.

The scientific and clinical challenges in developing a responsive closed-loop neurostimulation therapy for any brain disorder include identifying the anatomic targets in which to sense and stimulate and determining how to deliver and modulate the stimulation in response to clinical symptoms and physiologic biomarkers. These challenges have been addressed to a considerable extent for closed-loop responsive targeted neurostimulation for partial seizures. However, it seems certain that with additional understanding of the mechanisms of action of stimulation and with accumulating clinical experience, there will be further

advancements in the application of responsive neurostimulation as a treatment of epilepsy in general, and, specifically, with the application of the RNS System technology.

REFERENCES

1. Heck CN, King-Stephens D, Massey AD, et al. Two-year seizure reduction in adults with medically intractable partial onset epilepsy treated with responsive neurostimulation: final results of the RNS System Pivotal trial. Epilepsia 2014;55:432–41.
2. Bergey GK, Morrell MJ, Mizrahi EM, et al. Long-term treatment with responsive brain stimulation in adults with refractory partial seizures. Neurology 2015;84:810–7.
3. Meador KJ, Kapur R, Loring DW, et al. Quality of life and mood in patients with medically intractable epilepsy treated with targeted responsive neurostimulation. Epilepsy Behav 2015;45:242–7.
4. Loring DW, Kapur R, Meador KJ et al. Differential neuropsychological outcomes following targeted responsive neurostimulation for partial onset epilepsy. Epilepsia, in press. http://dx.doi.org/10.1111/epi.13191.
5. Weaver FM, Follett K, Stern M, et al. Bilateral deep brain stimulation vs best medical therapy for patients with advanced Parkinson disease: a randomized controlled trial. JAMA 2009;301:63–73.
6. Deuschl G, Schade-Brittinger C, Krack P, et al. A randomized trial of deep-brain stimulation for Parkinson's disease. N Engl J Med 2006;355:896–908.

7. Lyons KE, Pahwa R. Deep brain stimulation and essential tremor. J Clin Neurophysiol 2004;21:2–5.

8. Vidailhet M, Yelnik J, Lagrange C, et al. Bilateral pallidal deep brain stimulation for the treatment of patients with dystonia-choreoathetosis cerebral palsy: a prospective pilot study. Lancet Neurol 2009;8:709–17.

9. Kumar K, Taylor RS, Jacques L, et al. The effects of spinal cord stimulation in neuropathic pain are sustained: a 24-month follow-up of the prospective randomized controlled multicenter trial of the effectiveness of spinal cord stimulation. Neurosurgery 2008;63:762–70.

10. Fisher R, Salanova V, Witt T, et al. Electrical stimulation of the anterior nucleus of thalamus for treatment of refractory epilepsy. Epilepsia 2010; 51:899–908.

11. Salanova V, Witt T, Worth R, et al. Long-term efficacy and safety of thalamic stimulation for drug-resistant partial epilepsy. Neurology 2015;84:1017–25.

12. Hebb AO, Zhang JJ, Mahoor MH, et al. Creating the feedback loop: closed-loop neurostimulation. Neurosurg Clin N Am 2014;25:187–204.

13. Rosin B, Slovik M, Mitelman R, et al. Closed-loop deep brain stimulation is superior in ameliorating parkinsonism. Neuron 2011;72:370–84.

14. Wingeier B, Tcheng T, Koop MM, et al. Intra-operative STN DBS attenuates the prominent beta rhythm in the STN in Parkinson's disease. Exp Neurol 2006; 197:244–51.

15. Eusebio A, Thevathasan W, Doyle GL, et al. Deep brain stimulation can suppress pathological synchronisation in parkinsonian patients. J Neurol Neurosurg Psychiatry 2011;82:569–73.

16. Kuhn AA, Kempf F, Brucke C, et al. High-frequency stimulation of the subthalamic nucleus suppresses oscillatory beta activity in patients with Parkinson's disease in parallel with improvement in motor performance. J Neurosci 2008;28:6165–73.

17. Little S, Pogosyan A, Neal S, et al. Adaptive deep brain stimulation in advanced Parkinson disease. Ann Neurol 2013;74:449–57.

18. Little S, Brown P. What brain signals are suitable for feedback control of deep brain stimulation in Parkinson's disease? Ann N Y Acad Sci 2012;1265: 9–24.

19. Kwan P, Arzimanoglou A, Berg AT, et al. Definition of drug resistant epilepsy: consensus proposal by the ad hoc Task Force of the ILAE Commission on Therapeutic Strategies. Epilepsia 2010;51:1069–77.

20. Engel J Jr, Wiebe S, French J, et al. Practice parameter: temporal lobe and localized neocortical resections for epilepsy: report of the Quality Standards Subcommittee of the American Academy of Neurology, in association with the American Epilepsy Society and the American Association of Neurological Surgeons. Neurology 2003;60:538–47.

21. Wiebe S, Blume WT, Girvin JP, et al. A randomized, controlled trial of surgery for temporal-lobe epilepsy. N Engl J Med 2001;345:311–8.

22. Spencer SS, Berg AT, Vickrey BG, et al. Predicting long-term seizure outcome after resective epilepsy surgery: the multicenter study. Neurology 2005;65: 912–8.

23. VNS Therapy System Physicians Manual. Cyberonics, Inc. Available at: http://us.cyberonics.com/en/vns-therapy-for-epilepsy/healthcare-professionals/vns-therapy/manuals-page/. Accessed July 30, 2015.

24. Handforth A, DeGiorgio CM, Schachter SC, et al. Vagus nerve stimulation therapy for partial-onset seizures: a randomized active-control trial. Neurology 1998;51:48–55.

25. The Vagus Nerve Stimulation Study Group. A randomized controlled trial of chronic vagus nerve stimulation for treatment of medically intractable seizures. Neurology 1995;45:224–30.

26. Morris GL III, Mueller WM. Long-term treatment with vagus nerve stimulation in patients with refractory epilepsy. The Vagus Nerve Stimulation Study Group E01-E05. Neurology 1999;53:1731–5.

27. Ben-Menachem E, Manon-Espaillat R, Ristanovic R, et al. Vagus nerve stimulation for treatment of partial seizures: 1. A controlled study of effect on seizures. First International Vagus Nerve Stimulation Study Group. Epilepsia 1994;35:616–26.

28. Bergey GK. Neurostimulation in the treatment of epilepsy. Exp Neurol 2013;244:87–95.

29. Cooper IS, Amin I, Riklan M, et al. Chronic cerebellar stimulation in epilepsy. Clinical and anatomical studies. Arch Neurol 1976;33:559–70.

30. Chkhenkeli SA, Chkhenkeli IS. Effects of therapeutic stimulation of nucleus caudatus on epileptic electrical activity of brain in patients with intractable epilepsy. Stereotact Funct Neurosurg 1997; 69:221–4.

31. Chkhenkeli SA, Sramka M, Lortkipanidze GS, et al. Electrophysiological effects and clinical results of direct brain stimulation for intractable epilepsy. Clin Neurol Neurosurg 2004;106:318–29.

32. Sramka M, Fritz G, Gajdosova D, et al. Central stimulation treatment of epilepsy. Acta Neurochir Suppl (Wien) 1980;30:183–7.

33. Velasco F, Velasco M, Ogarrio C, et al. Electrical stimulation of the centromedian thalamic nucleus in the treatment of convulsive seizures: a preliminary report. Epilepsia 1987;28:421–30.

34. Fisher RS, Uematsu S, Krauss GL, et al. Placebo-controlled pilot study of centromedian thalamic stimulation in treatment of intractable seizures. Epilepsia 1992;33:841–51.

35. Chabardes S, Kahane P, Minotti L, et al. Deep brain stimulation in epilepsy with particular reference to the subthalamic nucleus. Epileptic Disord 2002;4: S83–93.

36. Vonck K, Boon P, Achten E, et al. Long-term amygdalohippocampal stimulation for refractory temporal lobe epilepsy. Ann Neurol 2002;52:556–65.

37. Tellez-Zentano JF, McLachlan RS, Parrent A, et al. Hippocampal electrical stimulation in mesial temporal lobe epilepsy. Neurology 2006;66(10):1490–4.

38. Velasco AL, Velasco F, Velasco M, et al. Electrical stimulation of the hippocampal epileptic foci for seizure control: a double-blind, long-term follow-up study. Epilepsia 2007;48:1895–903.

39. Penfield W, Jasper H. Electrocorticography. In: Epilepsy and the functional anatomy of the human brain. Boston: Little, Brown; 1954. p. 692–738.

40. Lesser RP, Kim SH, Beyderman L, et al. Brief bursts of pulse stimulation terminate afterdischarges caused by cortical stimulation. Neurology 1999;53:2073–81.

41. Motamedi GK, Lesser RP, Miglioretti DL, et al. Optimizing parameters for terminating cortical afterdischarges with pulse stimulation. Epilepsia 2002;43:836–46.

42. Osorio I, Frei MG, Sunderam S, et al. Automated seizure abatement in humans using electrical stimulation. Ann Neurol 2005;57:258–68.

43. Peters TE, Bhavaraju NC, Frei MG, et al. Network system for automated seizure detection and contingent delivery of therapy. J Clin Neurophysiol 2001;18:545–9.

44. Kossoff EH, Ritzl EK, Politsky JM, et al. Effect of an external responsive neurostimulator on seizures and electrographic discharges during subdural electrode monitoring. Epilepsia 2004;45:1560–7.

45. U.S. Department of Health and Human Services, Food and Drug Administration. RNS system, summary of safety and effectiveness, P100026. Available at: www.accessdata.fda.gov/cdrh_docs/pdf10/p100026b.pdf. Accessed August 14, 2014.

46. Sun FT, Morrell MJ. Closed-loop neurostimulation: the clinical experience. Neurotherapeutics 2014;11(3):553–63.

47. Morrell MJ, RNS System in Epilepsy Study Group. Responsive cortical stimulation for the treatment of medically intractable partial epilepsy. Neurology 2011;77:1295–304.

48. Engel J Jr, McDermott MP, Wiebe S, et al. Early surgical therapy for drug-resistant temporal lobe epilepsy: a randomized trial. JAMA 2012;307:922–30.

49. Markand ON, Salanova V, Whelihan E, et al. Health-related quality of life outcome in medically refractory epilepsy treated with anterior temporal lobectomy. Epilepsia 2000;41:749–59.

50. Spencer SS, Berg AT, Vickrey BG, et al. Health-related quality of life over time since resective epilepsy surgery. Ann Neurol 2007;62:327–34.

51. Riley TL, Porter RJ, White BG, et al. The hospital experience and seizure control. Neurology 1981;31:912–5.

52. Katariwala NM, Bakay RA, Pennell PB, et al. Remission of intractable partial epilepsy following implantation of intracranial electrodes. Neurology 2001;57:1505–7.

53. Dolezalova I, Brazdil M, Hermanova M, et al. Effect of partial drug withdrawal on the lateralization of interictal epileptiform discharges and its relationship to surgical outcome in patients with hippocampal sclerosis. Epilepsy Res 2014;108:1406–16.

54. Engel J Jr, Crandall PH. Falsely localizing ictal onsets with depth EEG telemetry during anticonvulsant withdrawal. Epilepsia 1983;24:344–55.

55. Marciani MG, Gotman J, Andermann F, et al. Patterns of seizure activation after withdrawal of antiepileptic medication. Neurology 1985;35:1537–43.

56. Marks DA, Katz A, Scheyer R, et al. Clinical and electrographic effects of acute anticonvulsant withdrawal in epileptic patients. Neurology 1991;41:508–12.

57. Lempka SF, Miocinovic S, Johnson MD, et al. In vivo impedance spectroscopy of deep brain stimulation electrodes. J Neural Eng 2009;6:046001.

58. Fong JS, Alexopoulos AV, Bingaman WE, et al. Pathologic findings associated with invasive EEG monitoring for medically intractable epilepsy. Am J Clin Pathol 2012;138:506–10.

59. Wei XF, Grill WM. Impedance characteristics of deep brain stimulation electrodes in vitro and in vivo. J Neural Eng 2009;6:046008.

60. Sillay KA, Rutecki P, Cicora K, et al. Long-term measurement of impedance in chronically implanted depth and subdural electrodes during responsive neurostimulation in humans. Brain Stimul 2013;6(5):718–26.

61. Moss J, Ryder T, Aziz TZ, et al. Electron microscopy of tissue adherent to explanted electrodes in dystonia and Parkinson's disease. Brain 2004;127:2755–63.

62. Stephan CL, Kepes JJ, SantaCruz K, et al. Spectrum of clinical and histopathologic responses to intracranial electrodes: from multifocal aseptic meningitis to multifocal hypersensitivity-type meningovasculitis. Epilepsia 2001;42:895–901.

63. King-Stephens D, Mirro E, Weber PB, et al. Lateralization of mesial temporal lobe epilepsy with chronic ambulatory electrocorticography. Epilepsia 2015;56:959–67.

Neuromodulation for Epilepsy

Vibhor Krishna, MD, SM[a], Francesco Sammartino, MD[a], Nicholas Kon Kam King, MD, PhD[b],
Rosa Qui Yue So, PhD[c], Richard Wennberg, MD, PhD[d],*

KEYWORDS

- Deep brain stimulation (DBS) • Intractable • Neurostimulation • Refractory seizures
- Trigeminal nerve stimulation (TNS) • Vagus nerve stimulation (VNS)

KEY POINTS

- Several neuromodulation options are available as palliative treatments for patients with medically refractory epilepsy.
- Vagus nerve stimulation, thalamic deep brain stimulation, and trigeminal nerve stimulation are currently the dominant nonresponsive treatment modalities in use.
- These different neurostimulation modalities all have a good safety profile and satisfactory rates of seizure reduction.

INTRODUCTION

A significant proportion of epilepsy patients is medically refractory,[1,2] and apart from those who are candidates for resective surgery, most will continue to have disabling seizures for rest of their lives.[3,4] Neuromodulation, or neurostimulation, is a palliative treatment option for many of these patients who are not eligible for resective surgery or who have persistent medically intractable refractory seizures despite previous epilepsy surgery.[5] Patients typically have partial onset seizures, with or without secondary generalization, or less frequently, generalized epilepsies. Candidates for neuromodulation usually have a long-standing history of intractable epilepsy and have undergone extensive investigations, including video-electroencephalography (EEG), advanced neuroimaging, and even intracranial subdural or depth electrode implantations for seizure localization in many cases. Most of these patients have been found to have no single discrete seizure onset localization; a minority has seizure onsets localized to nonresectable areas of eloquent cortex, for example, within the boundaries of language centers in the dominant temporal or frontal lobes.

Neuromodulation as an alternate form of treatment for intractable epilepsy was first considered based on historical observations that electrical stimulation of subcortical structures could modify the cortical EEG: high-frequency stimulation "desynchronized" the EEG and low-frequency stimulation "synchronized" the EEG.[6-9] Increased cortical synchrony mediated by low-frequency stimulation was demonstrated to be proepileptic, while cortical desynchronization mediated by high-frequency stimulation was shown to be antiepileptic.[10,11] Experimental or clinical antiepileptic

Conflicts of Interest: None.
Funding Source: None.
[a] Division of Neurosurgery, University of Toronto, Toronto Western Hospital, 399 Bathurst Street, Toronto, Ontario M5T2S8, Canada; [b] Department of Neurosurgery, National Neuroscience Institute, 11 Jalan Tan Tock Seng, Singapore 308433; [c] Department of Neural & Biomedical Technology, Institute for Infocomm Research, Agency for Science, Technology and Research, 1 Fusionopolis Way, #21-01 Connexis, Singapore 138632; [d] Division of Neurology, University of Toronto, Krembil Neuroscience Centre, University Health Network, Toronto Western Hospital, 399 Bathurst Street, Toronto, Ontario M5T2S8, Canada
* Corresponding author.
E-mail address: richard.wennberg@uhn.ca

Neurosurg Clin N Am 27 (2016) 123–131
http://dx.doi.org/10.1016/j.nec.2015.08.010
1042-3680/16/$ – see front matter © 2016 Elsevier Inc. All rights reserved.

properties were subsequently reported with chronic electrical stimulation of several different central and peripheral nervous system sites, including the cerebellum, hypothalamus (mamillary nuclei), vagus nerve, trigeminal nerve, caudate nucleus, substantia nigra, centromedian thalamus, anterior thalamus, subthalamic nucleus, and the amygdalohippocampal region.[12–44] In 1997, peripheral vagus nerve stimulation (VNS) was the first neurostimulation modality to be licensed for the treatment of patients with refractory epilepsy: controlled trials and subsequent widespread clinical usage have demonstrated significant, albeit modest, reduction in seizure frequencies.[45,46]

Following the successes of VNS, and with the hope that direct stimulation of central nervous system structures might provide additional, more robust, benefit in terms of seizure control, interest was renewed in performing clinical trials of deep brain stimulation (DBS) for epilepsy. The initial clinical trials of DBS in epilepsy were performed in the 1970s and 1980s, mainly using cerebellar and, to a lesser extent, thalamic or caudate stimulation.[12–16,21] DBS of the centromedian thalamic nucleus (CM) for intractable epilepsy was reported in several articles, with benefits in seizure control described in a most patients.[22–25,29]

The mechanisms by which DBS may control seizures are largely hypothetical and unproven. CM stimulation, acting via the widely projecting nonspecific thalamic system, is hypothesized to act through induction of cortical desynchronization, preventing seizure propagation and generalization.[22,29] Based on experimental data describing a "nigral control of epilepsy" system in rodents, controlled in large part by activity in the substantia nigra pars reticulata (SNpr),[47] subthalamic nucleus stimulation has been proposed to act through disfacilitation of SNpr neurons,[33] although there is no direct evidence for such a control system in primates. The anterior thalamus has been demonstrated to be involved in seizure propagation, both experimentally and clinically, and stimulation or lesioning of the anterior nucleus (AN) or its afferent pathways have been shown experimentally to have antiepileptic properties.[13,17–21] The dorsomedial nucleus of the thalamus, situated posterior and inferior to AN, has also been shown to be involved in the maintenance and propagation of seizures, specifically those involving limbic brain structures.[48,49] Anterior thalamus stimulation, aimed especially at AN, is thus hypothesized to act through blockade of corticothalamic synchrony, similar to CM. All of these proposed mechanisms are strictly hypothetical and, in fact, even the local effects of DBS are poorly understood. In a broad sense, most of the clinical effects of DBS can be considered to result from local inhibition of function, in that the effects are typically mimicked by lesions or application of inhibitory neurochemicals. Nevertheless, the mechanisms of local inhibition are unresolved, and it is possible that some effects of DBS could result from local neuronal or axonal excitation.

The exact parameters necessary to optimally alter the relevant corticothalamic networks with electrical stimulation are unknown, apart from the need for high-frequency stimulation (eg, $\geq$100 Hz). In the experimental models cited above, it is only high-frequency stimulation that shows antiepileptic properties, usually attributed to a cortical desynchronizing effect. In contrast, low-frequency stimulation tends to be proepileptic in experimental models, an observation conceptually linked to the increased synchronization in cortex that can be demonstrated through induction of the so-called recruiting rhythm with low-frequency thalamic stimulation.[6,10,11,50]

In general, neuromodulation therapies have excellent safety profiles, and stimulation can, at least theoretically, be titrated to optimize seizure control. However, neuromodulation is not expected to provide freedom from seizures or antiepileptic medications. The aim of these palliative treatment modalities is to either reduce seizure frequency or prevent secondary generalization in order to minimize the many risks associated with intractable epilepsy. At present, the primary neuromodulation modalities in use for the treatment of patients with medically refractory epilepsy are AN DBS, VNS, trigeminal nerve stimulation (TNS), and responsive neurostimulation (RNS) (**Fig. 1**).

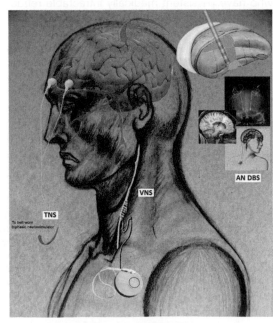

Fig. 1. Neuromodulation approaches.

The authors have not included RNS in this review because it is discussed elsewhere in this issue. In reviewing each of the main nonresponsive treatment modalities, a further brief historical perspective is offered, followed by the rationale of therapy and the clinical results to date.

ANTERIOR NUCLEUS DEEP BRAIN STIMULATION

Historically, Cooper and Upton[16] first reported on AN DBS for refractory complex partial seizures. In the subsequent decades, a small number of case series reported an acceptable efficacy and safety profile[35,37,38,42,43]: among the 19 total patients described in these pilot studies, there was a mean reduction in seizure frequency of 35% at 1 year (n = 19), 61% at 2 years (n = 13), and 65% in long-term follow-up (3–7 years; n = 14).[51] This mean reduction in seizure frequency paved the way for a large multicenter randomized trial: Stimulation of Anterior Nucleus of Thalamus for Epilepsy (SANTE),[52] which showed nearly identical results to those described in the collected pilot studies (**Table 1**). Currently, this procedure is approved for the treatment of refractory epilepsy in Europe and Canada but not in the United States.

Rationale

The AN forms part of the limbic circuit and is connected to the hippocampus via the mammillothalamic tract and the fornix.[59] This nucleus has abundant thalamocortical projections (to the cingulate gyrus, posterior parietal cortex, insular region, and lateral temporal cortex), making it an attractive target for modulation of seizure activity.[19,20,60] Combined EEG-functional MRI studies have shown involvement of the AN in the initiation and propagation of seizures in human idiopathic generalized epilepsy.[61,62] Mirski and colleagues[19,20,63] investigated seizure control after lesioning or electrical stimulation of the mammillothalamic tract or AN: in the pentylenetetrazol (PTZ) rat model, seizure threshold increased with high-frequency (but not low-frequency) stimulation of AN.[20] Similarly, in a sheep model of penicillin-induced epilepsy, only high-frequency stimulation reduced spontaneous and induced epileptic activity.[64] The mechanism underlying this efficacy of AN DBS could involve activation of the inhibitory corticothalamic projections.[65]

The implantation of electrodes for AN DBS is performed using frame-based stereotaxy.[66] In a parasagittal projection (4–5 mm from midline), the AN is located dorsal and anterior to the mammillothalamic tract. Intraoperative microelectrode recordings may aid electrode implantation by confirming the exit from the ventricle and entry into the thalamus.

Clinical Results

The early case series described acceptable safety profiles and benefits in seizure control in patients with various types of medically refractory epilepsy.[35,37,38,42,43,67] The reported mean seizure reduction rates varied between 50% and 90%. In the SANTE trial, 110 patients underwent implantation of DBS electrodes in the AN and were randomly assigned to stimulation ON (5 V, pulse width 90 μs, frequency 130 Hz, duty cycle 1 minute ON/5 minute OFF) or stimulation OFF for a 3-month blinded phase, after which all patients received AN stimulation (open-label phase). In the blinded phase, patients with active AN stimulation reported a 40% decrease in seizure frequency, versus a 15% decrease in the stimulation OFF group, a significant difference ($P = .002$). In long-term (5 year) follow-up, the mean reduction in seizure frequency was 69%, and 68% of patients reported 50% or better reduction in seizure frequency.[53] In the SANTE trial, AN DBS was well tolerated in most patients and unassociated with somatomotor side effects.[52,53] Memory disturbance was the most commonly reported side effect, likely related to stimulation-induced alterations in the circuit of Papez.[68]

VAGUS NERVE STIMULATION

Historically, the inhibition of motor activity by stimulation of vagal afferents was first reported in 1937 by Schweitzer and Wright.[69] Left VNS was approved by the US Food and Drug Administration (FDA) in 1997 for the treatment of medically refractory partial onset seizures.

Rationale

The vagus nerve is generally considered a parasympathetic nerve, but it also delivers sensations from the viscera. These visceral afferents project diffusely to cortex and subcortical regions, particularly the thalamus, via the medial reticular formation.[70,71] In patients with efficacious stimulation, decreased metabolic activity (assessed with technetium- hexamethylpropyleneamine oxime single-photon emission computed tomography) was observed bilaterally in the medial thalamus during the ON stimulation state.[71] VNS at clinically relevant parameters may also result in stimulation of unmyelinated C fibers (nociceptive fibers) leading to an arousal-like effect.[72,73] Zabara[72] studied VNS in canine models of strychnine -or PTZ-induced seizures. The stimulation (40 V, frequency 60 Hz, pulse width 0.6 ms) was

Table 1
Comparison of seizure control outcomes in clinical trials of different neuromodulation therapies

Modality	Patients (Refs.)	Responder Rate (>50% Seizure Reduction) 1 y, %	Responder Rate (>50% Seizure Reduction) 2 y, %	Responder Rate (>50% Seizure Reduction) Last Visit (y), %	Average Reduction in Seizure Frequency 1 y, %	Average Reduction in Seizure Frequency 2 y, %	Average Reduction in Seizure Frequency Last Visit (y), %
DBS (AN)	110[52,53]	43	54	68 (5)	41	56	69 (5)
VNS	65, 90[54,55]	44	59	64 (5)	36	52	56–66 (5) 76 (10)
TNS	35[56]	37	—	—	37	—	—
RNS	191, 230[57,58]	44	53	56–58 (3–6)	44	53	48–66(3–6)

Data from Refs.[52–58]

applied 1 to 3 minutes after the onset of motor seizure activity. The investigator reported a stimulation-induced interruption of seizure activity in a timely fashion (the longest interval observed was 14 seconds from the start of stimulation). The most effective parameters were intensity greater than 20 V, frequency higher than 20 Hz, and an approximate stimulus duration of 0.2 ms.[72] McLachlan,[73] using the penicillin seizure model in rats, reported a significant decrease in interictal spike activity, mean spike frequency, and amplitude with stimulation of the left vagus nerve. This effect persisted a few seconds after stimulation. Interestingly, a similar effect on spike frequency was seen in response to heating the rats' tails, suggesting that the antiepileptic effects of stimulation were not necessarily specific to the vagus nerve.[73] Chronic stimulation of the right vagal branch in a monkey model was also shown to reduce seizure frequency.[74] Clinically, however, the left vagus nerve is the preferred site of stimulation because it preferentially innervates the cardiac ventricles and is associated with a lesser risk of cardiac side effects.

Clinical Results

In a double-blind randomized controlled trial of VNS in a pediatric population (41 children with both localization-related and generalized epilepsy), the comparison groups were allocated to 2 different stimulation parameters: a treatment group: 0.25 mA, 30 Hz, 30 seconds ON/5 minutes OFF, and a control" group: 0.25 mA, 1 Hz, 14 seconds ON/60 minutes OFF.[75] After the initial phase, the first group received stimulation at the maximum tolerated current (maximum 1.75 mA), whereas in the second, control group, the output current was initially increased during the clinic visit but was then switched back to 0.25 mA at discharge. After the 20-week observation period, an overall reduction in seizure frequency and severity was observed as compared with baseline, without a statistically significant difference between the treatment and control groups. In a slightly different strategy, a large multicenter randomized trial (E03; 114 adult patients enrolled from 17 institutions) evaluated the effects of chronic stimulation and also the on-demand magnet activation strategy of the VNS device by instructing patients to activate the device during an aura.[45] The participants received 2 different stimulation parameters: high stimulation group: up to 3 mA, 20–50 Hz, 500 μs, ON 30–90 s/OFF 5–10 - minutes, and low stimulation group: up to 2.75 mA, 1 Hz, 130 μs, ON 30 s/OFF 60–180 minutes. After 14 weeks of stimulation, a significantly higher reduction in mean seizure frequency was

observed in the high-stimulation group (24% vs 6%, $P = .01$). Another large randomized trial of chronic stimulation involving 196 patients (E05) with similar study parameters was associated with a greater reduction in seizure frequency in the high-stimulation group (28% vs 15%, $P<.05$), especially among patients with complex partial seizures.[46] Regarding the effectiveness of the magnet intervention (ie, patient-controlled activation of the device near seizure onset), most patients thought the on-demand intervention to be effective, although there was no difference in reported efficacy between patient groups assigned to true activation versus sham activation (device programmed to 0 mA for magnet activation in the latter group).

The VNS surgical procedure carries a relatively low risk.[76] Common stimulation-related side effects (eg, cough, voice alteration, throat paresthesias) are typically mild and can be reversed by adjusting the stimulation parameters. The long-term follow-up data reveal a persistent benefit in seizure control that, similar to AN DBS, has been reported to gradually improve over time (see **Table 1**).[54,55]

TRIGEMINAL NERVE STIMULATION

Following the benefits in seizure control seen with invasive stimulation of the vagus nerve, and consistent with some of the aforementioned evidence suggesting a neuroanatomical nonspecificity to at least some of the effects of neuromodulation, the trigeminal nerve has been studied as a potential noninvasive alternative for peripheral nerve stimulation.[77] TNS may be delivered noninvasively due to the ease of stimulating trigeminal sensory roots within the facial tissue (eg, ophthalmic nerve, supratrochlear nerve, infraorbital nerve). Similar to AN DBS, this therapy is approved in Europe and Canada and is currently being investigated for FDA approval in the United States.

Rationale

Like VNS, TNS is also thought to generate an arousal-like effect from stimulation of the reticular activating system. Fanselow and colleagues[32] stimulated the infraorbital nerve bilaterally in 8 PTZ-induced epileptic rats. The stimulation (3–11 mA, 1–333 Hz) was delivered either continuously (60 seconds ON/60 seconds OFF duty cycle) or at the start of the seizure. The authors reported a reduction in seizure frequency with higher intensities (up to 7 mA) and frequencies (up to 100 Hz). Bilateral TNS yielded the same efficacy with slightly lower stimulation intensity.

Clinical Outcomes

In a pilot study, 2 patients with chronic intractable epilepsy received transcutaneous TNS over the infraorbital foramen.[78] The stimulation (8–25 mA, 120 Hz, 20–30 seconds ON/20–30 seconds OFF duty cycle) was well tolerated, and at 6 months both patients experienced a reduction in seizure frequency of up to 40%. In a case series of 13 patients presented by the same investigators, a mean reduction in seizure frequency of 59% was reported at 12 months.[78] A subsequent phase II randomized active control trial involving 42 patients with refractory epilepsy used bilateral TNS applied to the ophthalmic and supratrochlear nerves.[79] The treatment group received stimulation at 120 Hz, whereas the control group received stimulation at 2 Hz with a 2-second ON/90-second OFF duty cycle. Both groups were evaluated for 18 weeks and were stimulated for at least 12 hours per day. The investigators reported a responder rate (>50% reduction in seizure frequency) of 40% for the treatment group at 18 weeks, although the between-group difference was not statistically significant. No major device or stimulation-induced adverse events were reported. A long-term open-label follow-up of the patients in the phase II trial reported median reductions in seizure frequency in the treatment group of 27% at 6 months and 35% at 12 months (see **Table 1**), with 12-month responder rates of 37% for the treatment group and 31% for all subjects.[56]

SUMMARY

At present, several neuromodulation options are available for patients with refractory epilepsy. These modalities are currently adjunctive, palliative treatment options, but all have a good safety profile and acceptable rates of seizure reduction. The similarities in seizure control rates between the different treatment modalities currently in use (and others previously studied) are noteworthy (see **Table 1**) and suggest that stimulation-related perturbations of the nervous system in any of a variety of sites might have similar beneficial effects.[51] It is interesting to note that preliminary reports have recently described improved seizure control in response to yet another neuromodulation modality: noninvasive transcutaneous auricular (ear) stimulation,[57,80] presumably through activation of the auricular branch of the vagus nerve.[58]

Ongoing challenges in neuromodulation for epilepsy include an inability to accurately predict long-term outcomes at the level of the individual, and an inability to formulate management protocols that would assign specific neuromodulation modalities to different patient care scenarios. Likewise, identifying optimal patient-specific stimulation parameters remains for the most part a matter of trial and error. Future research in responsive neuromodulation therapies, where stimulation is given only in response to seizure detection, holds promise,[81] although the objective results of VNS magnet activation are sobering in this regard. Pivotal trial results from the first implantable RNS system have demonstrated similar beneficial effects on seizure control to those obtained with the nonresponsive neuromodulation modalities (see **Table 1**),[82,83] suggesting that all of the neurostimulation therapies available at this point in time may be considered potentially useful, although still suboptimal, treatment options for medically intractable epilepsy.

REFERENCES

1. Kwan P, Brodie MJ. Early identification of refractory epilepsy. N Engl J Med 2000;342:314–9.
2. Banerjee PN, Filippi D, Allen Hauser W. The descriptive epidemiology of epilepsy–a review. Epilepsy Res 2009;85:31–45.
3. Engel J Jr, Wiebe S, French J, et al. Practice parameter: temporal lobe and localized neocortical resections for epilepsy: report of the Quality Standards Subcommittee of the American Academy of Neurology, in association with the American Epilepsy Society and the American Association of Neurological Surgeons. Neurology 2003;60:538–47.
4. Loring DW, Meador KJ, Lee GP. Determinants of quality of life in epilepsy. Epilepsy Behav 2004;5: 976–80.
5. Fisher RS, Velasco AL. Electrical brain stimulation for epilepsy. Nat Rev Neurol 2014;10:261–70.
6. Dempsey EW, Morison RS. The production of rhythmically recurrent cortical potentials after localized thalamic stimulation. Am J Physiol 1942;135:293–300.
7. Morison RS, Dempsey EW. A study of thalamocortical relations. Am J Physiol 1942;135:281–92.
8. Morison RS, Dempsey EW. Mechanisms of thalamocortical augmentation and repetition. Am J Physiol 1943;138:297–308.
9. Moruzzi G, Magoun HW. Brainstem reticular formation and activation of the EEG. Electroencephalogr Clin Neurophysiol 1949;1:455–73.
10. Jasper HH, Droogleever-Fortuyn J. Experimental studies on the functional anatomy of petit mal epilepsy. Res Publ Assoc Res Nerv Ment Dis 1947;26: 272–98.
11. Hunter J, Jasper HH. Effects of thalamic stimulation in unanesthetized animals. The arrest reaction and petit mal seizure activation patterns and generalized convulsions. Electroencephalogr Clin Neurophysiol 1949;1:305–24.

12. Cooper IS, Amin I, Riklin M, et al. Chronic cerebellar stimulation in epilepsy. Clinical and anatomical studies. Arch Neurol 1976;33:559–70.

13. Cooper IS, Upton AR, Amin I. Reversibility of chronic neurologic deficits. Some effects of electrical stimulation of the thalamus and internal capsule in man. Appl Neurophysiol 1980;43:244–58.

14. Sramka M, Fritz G, Galanda M, et al. Some observations in treatment stimulation of epilepsy. Acta Neurochir 1976;(Suppl 23):257–62.

15. Wright GD, McLellan DL, Brice JG. A double-blind trial of chronic cerebellar stimulation in twelve patients with severe epilepsy. J Neurol Neurosurg Psychiatry 1984;47:769–74.

16. Cooper IS, Upton ARM. Therapeutic implications of modulation of metabolism and functional activity of cerebral cortex by chronic stimulation of cerebellum and thalamus. Biol Psychiatry 1985;20:809–11.

17. Mirski MA, Ferrendelli JA. Anterior thalamic mediation of generalized pentylenetetrazol seizures. Brain Res 1986;399:212–23.

18. Mirski MA, Ferrendelli JA. Interruption of the connections of the mammillary bodies protects against generalized pentylenetetrazol seizures in guinea pigs. J Neurosci 1987;7:662–70.

19. Mirski MA, Fisher RS. Electrical stimulation of the mammillary nuclei increases seizure threshold to pentylenetetrazol in rats. Epilepsia 1994;35:1309–16.

20. Mirski MA, Rossell LA, Terry JB, et al. Anticonvulsant effect of anterior thalamic high frequency electrical stimulation in the rat. Epilepsy Res 1997;28:89–100.

21. Upton ARM, Amin I, Garnett S, et al. Evoked metabolic responses in the limbic-striate system produced by stimulation of anterior thalamic nucleus in man. Pacing Clin Electrophysiol 1987;10:217–25.

22. Velasco F, Velasco M, Ogarrio C, et al. Electrical stimulation of the centromedian thalamic nucleus in the treatment of convulsive seizures: a preliminary report. Epilepsia 1987;28:421–30.

23. Velasco M, Velasco F, Velasco AL, et al. Epileptiform EEG activities of the centromedian thalamic nuclei in patients with intractable partial motor, complex partial, and generalized seizures. Epilepsia 1989;30:295–306.

24. Velasco F, Velasco M, Velasco AL, et al. Effect of chronic electrical stimulation of the centromedian thalamic nuclei on various intractable seizure patterns: I. Clinical seizures and paroxysmal EEG activity. Epilepsia 1993;34:1052–64.

25. Velasco F, Velasco M, Velasco AL, et al. Electrical stimulation of the centromedian thalamic nucleus in control of seizures: long-term studies. Epilepsia 1995;36:63–71.

26. Velasco M, Velasco F, Velasco AL, et al. Subacute electrical stimulation of the hippocampus blocks intractable temporal lobe seizures and paroxysmal EEG activities. Epilepsia 2000;41:158–69.

27. Velasco F, Carrillo-Ruiz JD, Brito F, et al. Double-blind, randomized controlled pilot study of bilateral cerebellar stimulation for treatment of intractable motor seizures. Epilepsia 2005;46:1071–81.

28. Velasco AL, Velasco F, Velasco M, et al. Electrical stimulation of the hippocampal epileptic foci for seizure control: a double-blind, long-term follow-up study. Epilepsia 2007;48:1895–903.

29. Fisher RS, Uematsu S, Krauss GL, et al. Placebo-controlled pilot study of centromedian thalamic stimulation in treatment of intractable seizures. Epilepsia 1992;33:841–51.

30. Chkhenkeli SA, Chkhenkeli IS. Effects of therapeutic stimulation of nucleus caudatus on epileptic electrical activity of brain in patients with intractable epilepsy. Stereotact Funct Neurosurg 1997;69:221–4.

31. Vercueil L, Benazzouz A, Deransart C, et al. High frequency stimulation of the sub-thalamic nucleus suppresses absence seizures in the rat: comparison with neurotoxic lesions. Epilepsy Res 1998;31:39–46.

32. Fanselow EE, Reid AP, Nicolelis MA. Reduction of pentylenetetrazol-induced seizure activity in awake rats by seizure-triggered trigeminal nerve stimulation. J Neurosci 2000;20:8160–8.

33. Loddenkemper T, Pan A, Neme S, et al. Deep brain stimulation in epilepsy. J Clin Neurophysiol 2001;18:514–32.

34. Chabardès S, Kahane P, Minotti L, et al. Deep brain stimulation in epilepsy with particular reference to the subthalamic nucleus. Epileptic Disord 2002;4(Suppl 3):83–93.

35. Hodaie M, Wennberg RA, Dostrovsky JO, et al. Chronic anterior thalamic stimulation for intractable epilepsy. Epilepsia 2002;43:603–8.

36. Vonck K, Boon P, Achten E, et al. Long-term amygdalohippocampal stimulation for refractory temporal lobe epilepsy. Ann Neurol 2002;52:556–65.

37. Kerrigan JF, Litt B, Fisher RS, et al. Electrical stimulation of the anterior nucleus of the thalamus for the treatment of intractable epilepsy. Epilepsia 2004;45:346–54.

38. Andrade DM, Zumsteg D, Hamani C, et al. Long-term follow-up of patients with thalamic deep brain stimulation for epilepsy. Neurology 2006;66:1571–3.

39. DiGiorgio CM, Shewmon A, Murray D, et al. Pilot study of trigeminal nerve stimulation (TNS) for epilepsy: a proof-of-concept trial. Epilepsia 2006;47:1213–5.

40. Tellez-Zenteno JF, McLachlan RS, Parrent A, et al. Hippocampal electrical stimulation in mesial temporal lobe epilepsy. Neurology 2006;66:1490–4.

41. Boon P, Vonck K, De Herdt V, et al. Deep brain stimulation in patients with refractory temporal lobe epilepsy. Epilepsia 2007;48:1551–60.

42. Lim S-N, Lee S-T, Tsai Y-T, et al. Electrical stimulation of the anterior nucleus of the thalamus for intractable

epilepsy: a long-term follow-up study. Epilepsia 2007;48:342–7.

43. Osorio I, Overman J, Giftakis J, et al. High frequency thalamic stimulation for inoperable mesial temporal lobe epilepsy. Epilepsia 2007;48:1561–71.

44. Vesper J, Steinhoff B, Rona S, et al. Chronic high frequency deep brain stimulation of the STN/SNr for progressive myoclonic epilepsy. Epilepsia 2007;48: 1984–9.

45. A randomized controlled trial of chronic vagus nerve stimulation for treatment of medically intractable seizures. The Vagus Nerve Stimulation Study Group. Neurology 1995;45:224–30.

46. Handforth A, DeGiorgio CM, Schachter SC, et al. Vagus nerve stimulation therapy for partial-onset seizures. A randomized active-control trial. Neurology 1998;51:48–55.

47. Iadarola MJ, Gale K. Substantia nigra: site of anticonvulsant activity mediated by gamma-aminobutyric acid. Science 1982;218:1237–40.

48. Bertram EH, Zhang DX, Mangan P, et al. Functional anatomy of limbic epilepsy: a proposal for central synchronization of a diffusely hyperexcitable network. Epilepsy Res 1998;32:194–205.

49. Bertram EH, Mangan PS, Zhang D, et al. The midline thalamus: alterations and a potential role in limbic epilepsy. Epilepsia 2001;42:967–78.

50. Zumsteg D, Lozano AM, Wennberg RA. Rhythmic cortical EEG synchronization with low frequency stimulation of the anterior and medial thalamus for epilepsy. Clin Neurophysiol 2006;117:2272–8.

51. Wennberg R. Chronic anterior thalamic deep-brain stimulation as a treatment for intractable epilepsy. In: Schelter B, Timmer J, Schulze-Bonhage A, editors. Seizure prediction in epilepsy. Weinheim (Germany): Wiley-VCH; 2008. p. 307–16.

52. Fisher R, Salanova V, Witt T, et al. Electrical stimulation of the anterior nucleus of thalamus for treatment of refractory epilepsy. Epilepsia 2010;51:899–908.

53. Salanova V, Witt T, Worth R, et al. Long-term efficacy and safety of thalamic stimulation for drug-resistant partial epilepsy. Neurology 2015;84:1017–25.

54. Elliott RE, Morsi A, Tanweer O, et al. Efficacy of vagus nerve stimulation over time: review of 65 consecutive patients with treatment-resistant epilepsy treated with VNS > 10 years. Epilepsy Behav 2011;20:478–83.

55. Kuba R, Brazdil M, Kalina M, et al. Vagus nerve stimulation: longitudinal follow-up of patients treated for 5 years. Seizure 2009;18:269–74.

56. Soss J, Heck C, Murray D, et al. A prospective long-term study of external trigeminal nerve stimulation for drug-resistant epilepsy. Epilepsy Behav 2015;42:44–7.

57. He W, Jing X, Wang X, et al. Transcutaneous auricular vagus nerve stimulation as a complementary therapy for pediatric epilepsy: a pilot trial. Epilepsy Behav 2013;28:343–6.

58. Clancy JA, Mary DA, Witte KK, et al. Non-invasive vagus nerve stimulation in healthy humans reduces sympathetic nerve activity. Brain Stimul 2014;7: 871–7.

59. Papez JW. A proposed mechanism of emotion. Arch Neurol Psychiatry 1937;38:725–43.

60. Child ND, Benarroch EE. Anterior nucleus of the thalamus: functional organization and clinical implications. Neurology 2013;81:1869–76.

61. Moeller F, Siebner HR, Wolff S, et al. Changes in activity of striato-thalamo-cortical network precede generalized spike wave discharges. Neuroimage 2008;39:1839–49.

62. Tyvaert L, Chassagnon S, Sadikot A, et al. Thalamic nuclei activity in idiopathic generalized epilepsy: an EEG-fMRI study. Neurology 2009;73:2018–22.

63. Mirski MA, Ferrendelli JA. Interruption of the mammillothalamic tract prevents seizures in guinea pigs. Science 1984;226:72–4.

64. Stypulkowski PH, Giftakis JE, Billstrom TM. Development of a large animal model for investigation of deep brain stimulation for epilepsy. Stereotact Funct Neurosurg 2011;89:111–22.

65. Molnar GF, Sailer A, Gunraj CA, et al. Changes in motor cortex excitability with stimulation of anterior thalamus in epilepsy. Neurology 2006;66:566–71.

66. Krishna V, Lozano AM. Brain stimulation for intractable epilepsy: anterior thalamus and responsive stimulation. Ann Indian Acad Neurol 2014;17:S95–8.

67. Lee KJ, Shon YM, Cho CB. Long-term outcome of anterior thalamic nucleus stimulation for intractable epilepsy. Stereotact Funct Neurosurg 2012; 90:379–85.

68. Hamani C, Dubiela FP, Soares JC, et al. Anterior thalamus deep brain stimulation at high current impairs memory in rats. Exp Neurol 2010;225:154–62.

69. Schweitzer A, Wright S. Effects on the knee jerk of stimulation of the central end of the vagus and of various changes in the circulation and respiration. J Physiol 1937;88:459–75.

70. Ko D, Heck C, Grafton S, et al. Vagus nerve stimulation activates central nervous system structures in epileptic patients during PET H2(15)O blood flow imaging. Neurosurgery 1996;39:426–30 [discussion: 430–1].

71. Ring HA, White S, Costa DC, et al. A SPECT study of the effect of vagal nerve stimulation on thalamic activity in patients with epilepsy. Seizure 2000;9:380–4.

72. Zabara J. Inhibition of experimental seizures in canines by repetitive vagal stimulation. Epilepsia 1992;33:1005–12.

73. McLachlan RS. Suppression of interictal spikes and seizures by stimulation of the vagus nerve. Epilepsia 1993;34:918–23.

74. Lockard JS, Congdon WC, DuCharme LL. Feasibility and safety of vagal stimulation in monkey model. Epilepsia 1990;31(Suppl 2):S20–6.

75. Klinkenberg S, Aalbers MW, Vles JS, et al. Vagus nerve stimulation in children with intractable epilepsy: a randomized controlled trial. Dev Med Child Neurol 2012;54:855–61.

76. Ben-Menachem E. Vagus nerve stimulation, side effects, and long-term safety. J Clin Neurophysiol 2001;18:415–8.

77. DeGiorgio CM, Shewmon DA, Whitehurst T. Trigeminal nerve stimulation for epilepsy. Neurology 2003; 61:421–2.

78. DeGiorgio CM, Murray D, Markovic D, et al. Trigeminal nerve stimulation for epilepsy: long-term feasibility and efficacy. Neurology 2009;72:936–8.

79. DeGiorgio CM, Soss J, Cook IA, et al. Randomized controlled trial of trigeminal nerve stimulation for drug-resistant epilepsy. Neurology 2013;80:786–91.

80. Stefan H, Kreiselmeyer G, Kerling F, et al. Transcutaneous vagus nerve stimulation (t-VNS) in pharmacoresistant epilepsies: a proof of concept trial. Epilepsia 2012;53:e115–8.

81. Osorio I, Frei MG, Sunderam S, et al. Automated seizure abatement in humans using electrical stimulation. Ann Neurol 2005;57:258–68.

82. Heck CN, King-Stephens D, Massey AD, et al. Two-year seizure reduction in adults with medically intractable partial onset epilepsy treated with responsive neurostimulation: final results of the RNS System Pivotal trial. Epilepsia 2014;55:432–41.

83. Bergey GK, Morrell MJ, Mizrahi EM, et al. Long-term treatment with responsive brain stimulation in adults with refractory partial seizures. Neurology 2015;84: 810–7.

Index

Note: Page numbers of article titles are in **boldface** type.

Neurosurg Clin N Am 27 (2016) 133–136
http://dx.doi.org/10.1016/S1042-3680(15)00111-4
1042-3680/16/$ – see front matter © 2016 Elsevier Inc. All rights reserved.

Moving?

Make sure your subscription moves with you!

To notify us of your new address, find your **Clinics Account Number** (located on your mailing label above your name), and contact customer service at:

Email: journalscustomerservice-usa@elsevier.com

800-654-2452 (subscribers in the U.S. & Canada)
314-447-8871 (subscribers outside of the U.S. & Canada)

Fax number: 314-447-8029

Elsevier Health Sciences Division
Subscription Customer Service
3251 Riverport Lane
Maryland Heights, MO 63043

*To ensure uninterrupted delivery of your subscription, please notify us at least 4 weeks in advance of move.

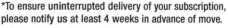

Moving?

Make sure your subscription moves with you!

To notify us of your new address, find your Clinics Account Number (located on your mailing label above your name), and contact customer service at:

Email: journalscustomerservice-usa@elsevier.com

800-654-2452 (subscribers in the U.S. & Canada)
314-447-8871 (subscribers outside of the U.S. & Canada)

Fax number: 314-447-8029

Elsevier Health Sciences Division
Subscription Customer Service
3251 Riverport Lane
Maryland Heights, MO 63043

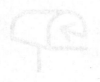

*To ensure uninterrupted delivery of your subscription, please notify us at least 4 weeks in advance of move.

Printed and bound by CPI Group (UK) Ltd, Croydon, CR0 4YY

03/10/2024

01040376-0014